Survey Responses

Survey Responses

An Evaluation of Their Validity

Ellen J. Wentland

Departments of Psychology and Psychiatry
Rush University
Chicago, Illinois
and
Department of Psychology
North Central College
Naperville, Illinois

with

Kent W. Smith

American Bar Foundation
Chicago, Illinois

Academic Press, Inc.
A Division of Harcourt Brace & Company
San Diego   New York   Boston   London   Sydney   Tokyo   Toronto

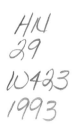

Academic Press, Inc.
1250 Sixth Avenue, San Diego, California 92101-4311

United Kingdom Edition published by
Academic Press Limited
24–28 Oval Road, London NW1 7DX

Library of Congress Cataloging-in Publication Data

Wentland, Ellen J.
    Survey responses : an evaluation of their validity / Ellen J.
Wentland, Kent W. Smith.
        p.   cm.
    Includes bibliographical references (p.   ) and index.
    ISBN 0-12-744030-5
    1. Social. surveys.   I. Smith, Kent W.   II. Title.
HN29.W423   1993
300'.72--dc20   92-46917
                                                              CIP

PRINTED IN THE UNITED STATES OF AMERICA
93 94 95 96 97 98   QW   9 8 7 6 5 4 3 2 1

Contents

Chapter 9. Meta-Analysis: Results and Discussion

Chapter 10. Meta-Analysis: Discussion and Integration

Chapter 11. Meta-Analysis: Summary and Conclusions

PART V   General Summary

Chapter 12. Summation and Conclusions   191

Preface

I participated in an American Bar Foundation research project on income tax noncompliance and evasion that began in 1984. It appeared that information on the prevalence of this behavior was often obtained from surveys. Further, information concerning the possible demographic, behavioral, and attitudinal correlates of noncompliance and evasion, important for behavioral prediction, model and theory building, and policy development, was also largely gleaned from surveys. Surveys, however, are based mainly on the self-reports of individuals. As such, I wondered, how much confidence could be placed in the findings?

What started as an interest in the degree of accuracy of responses to questions about compliance with income tax laws became a more general concern with the validity of survey responses to questions about behavior and personal characteristics. An investigation into the validity of survey responses to questions of this type might also contribute to our knowledge about the correlates or causes of response inaccuracy and suggest approaches to increase accuracy.

I decided that my questions would be best answered by examining studies that had evaluated the accuracy of individuals' responses to questions about behavior and personal characteristics, as opposed to investigating aggregate level validity. Forward and reverse record check studies represent attempts to determine the validity of individuals' responses to survey questions. An examination and analysis of these studies could provide information about the level of accuracy found in surveys, and perhaps that to be expected. Factors associated with response accuracy or inaccuracy, such as the question topic or the time frame of the question, might also be identified through this process and systematically evaluated.

As I reviewed the relevant literature, I found that there had been no previous attempt to pull together data from the many studies that had checked the accuracy of individuals' responses to survey questions about behavior and personal characteristics. Yet the question of the actual level of accuracy in surveys is extremely important, especially when we consider the high costs associated with implementing programs or developing policies based on erroneous data.

There was, however, an existing data base in the form of a number of individual studies on the subject. Locating these studies, reworking and reanalyzing the data presented so that comparisons across studies could be made, and identifying variables potentially affecting response accuracy presented a formidable task.

I believed, however, that much could be learned by taking an overview of these data. Researchers now turning to individual studies for information and guidance may be misled when certain nonobvious particulars of studies affect outcomes. Also, contrary findings to questions involving similar topics and methods create confusion. A systematic examination and quantitative assessment of these data in the aggregate, however, might reveal patterns and help explain inconsistencies and apparent contradictions.

My goals in writing this book were:

(1) to contribute to our knowledge about the level of accuracy in surveys through an intensive examination and analysis of the data from studies that have, using external criteria, evaluated the validity of individuals' responses to survey questions about behavior and personal characteristics;

(2) to identify variables associated with response accuracy, through an exploration of the studies included in this review and also through a consideration of other relevant research and theories;

(3) to contribute to our understanding of the causes of response error through a meta-analysis, whereby the factors appearing to affect response accuracy are systematically evaluated;

(4) to develop a theoretical perspective concerning the variables found to influence response accuracy; and

(5) to provide practical assistance to researchers involved in designing and interpreting surveys.

I believe that this book will be of interest to researchers working in the area of survey research or interested in the validity of self-reports in general. This would include social scientists, statisticians, and market researchers. Cognitive and social psychologists might be particularly interested in my work since I drew heavily on recent research and theories in those areas in the identification of variables to be included in the meta-analysis and in the interpretation of the results from this analysis.

This book would also be suitable for undergraduate or graduate level research methods courses. The qualitative analysis of the studies that I included is a review and critique of the research, often including a reanalysis or reinterpretation of the data. Students would benefit from reading the original reports and comparing these with my summaries and interpretations.

The meta-analysis is also carefully explained and would provide good background in meta-analytic techniques and regression analysis.

Information in this book should also be useful to practitioners involved in the design, implementation, and interpretation of surveys. Theoretical perspectives as well as practical guidelines are provided.

I gratefully acknowledge the financial support provided for this project by the American Bar Foundation. I also gratefully acknowledge the contributions of Kent W. Smith, Director of the Tax Compliance Research Project at the Foundation. The assistance and expertise that Kent provided in the meta-analysis phase of the research is especially appreciated.

The comments, insights, suggestions, and encouragement offered by Norman Bradburn, Robert Mason, and Seymour Sudman, who all reviewed earlier versions of the manuscript, are also sincerely appreciated.

Colleagues at the American Bar Foundation who participated in the item ratings and offered comments on parts of the manuscript, whose assistance I acknowledge gratefully, are Karyl Kinsey, Margaret Poethig, and Margaret Troha.

I also thank Margaret Poethig and Anne Hill for their help in preparing the tables and for their careful typing of earlier versions of parts of the manuscript.

Finally, I want to thank the editors at Academic Press, namely, Nikki Fine, Marianne Maggini, and Lori Asbury for their support and assistance in preparing this publication.

Ellen Wentland

Part I
Background of the Research

1

Introduction

Survey researchers have concluded that many factors influence individuals' responses to survey questions, thereby affecting the accuracy or truthfulness of their self-reports, even in so-called "matters of fact." A body of evidence from studies supports this conclusion.

Clarification of the meaning of certain terms used in this report is important. The words *accurate* and *truth* are not meant to imply intentionality. Some inaccurate or untruthful reporting by respondents may be unintentional, due to reasons such as confusion about the question asked, faulty memory, or distorted recall. For example, respondents may believe that they performed certain behaviors when they did not, simply because these beliefs are consistent with their self-image (Spanier, 1976; Cahalan, 1968).

Some inaccurate or untruthful reporting, of course, is intentional. Some possible motives for an untruthful or inaccurate response include concern regarding the social desirability of a response or a desire to answer questions according to perceived social expectations; unwillingness to provide information that may be incriminating or lead to sanctions; desire for personal status or ego enhancement; and felt need to present oneself as possessing particular characteristics, or as having behaved in certain ways, perhaps due to reference group identification.

Factors Affecting Response Validity

Some factors that have been investigated with respect to their effect on the accuracy of self-reports include the particular data-gathering approach used in the survey, as in Begin & Boivin (1980); anonymous versus identifiable self-reports, as in Malbin & Moskowitz (1983); question order, as in McFarland (1981); survey sponsorship, as in Seltzer (1983); interviewer characteristics and expectations, as in Singer, Frankel, & Glassman (1983); the period of time covered by a question, as in Gray (1955); the level of threat to the respondent posed by various types of questions or the sensitivity of the subject, as in Locander, Sudman, & Bradburn (1976); question wording, as in Mauldin & Marks (1950); and faulty recall, as in Spanier (1976).

Sudman & Bradburn (1974) used the term *response effect* to refer to the amount of error in the response to a question associated with a particular factor. They examined the principal sources and relative magnitudes of response effects in surveys through an extensive review and analysis of the survey literature to date.

Forty-six independent variables believed to be potential sources of response effects were identified for study in Sudman & Bradburn's (1974) research. These included variables associated with the interviewer role, such as the interviewer's social background characteristics; variables associated with the respondent's role, including characteristics and respondent role motivation; and variables associated with the task, such as the perceived social desirability of the answer. A measure was developed to assess the relative magnitude of the response effects associated with the particular variables within each study evaluated; then data were combined across studies. Sudman & Bradburn (1974) concluded that task variables seemed to be the most important factors related to response error overall.

Groves (1989) focused on the different perspectives taken by researchers from various fields toward the problem of survey errors. He discussed and attempted to consolidate the literatures as they related to different types of survey errors, including measurement errors, that is, "errors in data actually obtained by the survey" (p. 295). Groves noted that "cognitive processing appears to be central to survey measurement error" (p. 407).

Attempts to Estimate Response Validity

Aggregate-Level Comparisons

Assuming that various survey designs and procedures may produce different amounts of response error, researchers have compared results obtained from different approaches, for example, telephone versus face-to-face interviews, or varying question order. Frequently these surveys concerned sensitive or threatening subjects, such as respondents' involvement in illegal activities. In these studies, researchers often concluded that the best approach for measuring a particular subject was the approach that produced the most admissions. However, no reference was made to external criteria against which responses were compared. Therefore, the procedure or design that was actually associated with the highest level of accuracy could not be determined.

In other efforts to estimate the validity of survey measurements, research-ers compared aggregate level survey findings with data from other sources. These external data are believed to be accurate, or at least to represent an independent source of information gathered by means other than surveys. Gottfredson & Hindelang (1977), for example, compared data obtained from *National Crime Survey* victimization studies with crime statistics published in the Federal Bureau of Investigation's *Uniform Crime Reports*. As another example, Popham & Schmidt (1981) compared reported alcohol purchases with actual sales statistics.

In some cases, the external data come from other surveys. To the extent that similar findings are obtained from a variety of approaches and samples, researchers believe that they can have more confidence in their results and in the quality of their data. For example, Miller (1953) compared results obtained from preliminary tabulations of data from the 1950 U.S. Census with information obtained in the U.S. Census Bureau's Current Population Sur-vey. Miller concluded that the family income data from the two sources were comparable.

Another approach used to assess the accuracy of self-reports involves compar-ing the responses of persons in groups known to differ along some specific dimension. For example, Erickson & Empey (1963) argued for the accuracy of their interview data on delinquent behavior obtained from groups of young males since the data distinguished between those with at most one court appearance and those described as repeat or incarcerated offenders.

Although these types of comparisons are useful and important, they do not provide information regarding the accuracy of an individual's response. Ag-gregate data may reflect compensating errors that balance out. For exam-ple, in a survey of stock ownership, 20% of the respondents may claim to own stock when they do not, and 20% may deny owning stock when they do. The percentage of respondents claiming to own stock would reflect actual stock ownership, even though 40% of the respondents were not truthful. This misrepresentation of ownership would be especially problematic in an individual-level analysis, for example, in an examination of the characteristics of those who own and/or those who do not own stocks.

Validation of Individual Responses

A number of studies on a wide variety of topics using different designs, procedures, and samples have approached the problem of response error from the level of the individual respondent. Researchers were able to obtain information about the respondent from an outside source, either before (reverse record check) or after (forward record check) the survey. Indivi-duals' responses were then checked against these external criteria. In many of these studies, attempts were also made to determine the relationship between response inaccuracy and particular variables, for example, respondent characteristics.

Numerous topics have been included in these individual-level evaluations, including sensitive ones. Midanik (1982) reviewed studies of this type in the area of alcohol use, but apparently there has been no previous attempt to make an overall assessment of the levels of accuracy found in these research efforts and perhaps to be expected in surveys. Such an assessment would also permit the identification of factors potentially associated with higher levels of accuracy and a systematic, quantitative evaluation of these factors. This information would be useful for evaluating existing survey data and for designing future surveys.

Plan of This Book

The plan of this book is to review and analyze data from studies that have, through the use of external criteria, assessed the validity of individuals' responses to questions concerning personal characteristics and behavior in a wide variety of areas. In this endeavor, the two major goals are to determine the level of accuracy in responses to survey questions of this type, and to identify and systematically evaluate factors associated with response accuracy.

Six points need elaboration. First, although our data are subjected to a quantitative assessment in the form of a meta-analysis, the studies included in this report are first presented in a detailed, qualitative review. The presentation of this type of review is important for many reasons.

The studies that were selected for inclusion in this report are scattered over an approximate 40-year period, and most readers would probably only be familiar with a portion of this research. Further, some of the data included in this review are different from those presented in the original reports. In order to address the questions raised in this investigation and to enable comparisons across questions and studies, a considerable amount of reworking and reanalysis of data, or secondary analysis, was often necessary. In a very few instances, certain data were excluded for reasons such as inconsistencies in the reported number of cases, such that it was impossible to determine which group or groups were being measured. In other cases, personal communication with authors was helpful in obtaining clarification or additional information. The in-depth discussions of the original research reports will help the reader understand any apparent discrepancies.

The detailed discussion of these studies also allows the reader to follow the process of the identification of factors that may have affected response accuracy. In this effort, the interpretations and speculations of the primary researchers are often presented. These interpretations are important to consider because the primary researchers were closest to the data and the data-gathering effort. The studies included in this review are very diverse in terms of their goals, topics, designs, and subject populations. An exploration of the researchers' conclusions concerning the factors contributing to accuracy was one approach used to identify those variables that may be essential or common to all questions and surveys.

Often, however, the identification of variables affecting validity was not the focus of the primary researchers. At other times, potentially important factors were not discussed. Much of the interpretation and analysis of these studies in this regard, therefore, is our own.

Second, to insure a comprehensive data base for the quantitative analysis, it was important to include as many studies as possible in this report. The issue of survey data accuracy is best addressed by exploring as much of the available evidence as possible. When individual studies were reviewed, therefore, they were retained for analysis when we were reasonably confident in the criteria used to verify the accuracy of responses and when the data were presented in, or could be converted to, a form which allowed for comparability across studies. Further, rather than exclude certain otherwise appropriate studies or questions for such reasons as poor design or use of possibly inexact criteria, potential problems are discussed or noted in the text.[1]

Third, this investigation will focus solely on studies that have evaluated the accuracy of individuals' responses, as opposed to estimating validity through aggregate level comparisons. As previously discussed, the purpose of this review is not only to assess the level of response validity found in surveys, but also to identify and evaluate factors which appear to be associated with accurate responding. It is our intent to explore this association through a meta-analysis, whereby the relationship between survey and question characteristics, and the percentages of accurate responses to particular questions is systematically evaluated. This type of investigation required obtaining information about the accuracy of individuals' responses.

Fourth, this report includes only studies concerned with respondents' behavior or personal characteristics, as opposed to attitudes, since attitudinal data cannot be verified. Sudman & Bradburn (1974) referred to the variability,

---

[1]According to Glass (1976), "It is an empirical question whether relatively poorly designed studies give results significantly at variance with those of the best designed studies ... At any rate, I believe the difference to be so small that to integrate research results by eliminating the 'poorly done' studies is to discard a vast amount of important data" (p. 4). Sudman & Bradburn (1974) considered several factors in making judgments about the quality of the research studies included in their review. They found, however, that results weighted by the estimated quality of the studies did not differ from the unweighted results.

as opposed to the accuracy, of attitudinal reports. Other researchers have looked at the reliability or consistency of responses. However, the assessment of the accuracy of self-reports of attitudes remains problematic, since consistency does not necessarily equate with accuracy. Respondents' expressions of attitudes can logically be suspected of being strongly influenced by their self-presentation or social desirability concerns. Also, survey researchers have long been aware of the possibility that simply by asking respondents to state attitudes or to indicate agreement or disagreement with prespecified attitudinal statements, attitudes may be created, or at least expressed, where they did not formerly exist (Rosenberg, 1968; Hawkins & Coney, 1981).

Fifth, we included only those studies in which individuals' responses were validated through the use of external criteria, that is, information collected independently of the respondent. Further, external criteria were considered acceptable only if we had a reasonable amount of confidence in their accuracy. The use of official records as criteria met this test in many cases. At the same time, we recognize that many problems exist with respect to the accuracy of records, even official records, and that perhaps no criterion is 100% valid.

At times, concerns about criterion accuracy led us to exclude certain studies or portions of data from this analysis. Any concerns about the records or validating data used for response validation in the studies included herein are discussed in detail in the qualitative analysis.

In addition to possible problems with the accuracy of records, there is also potential for error in activities associated with checking responses against records or in recording data. The extent of these types of errors in the studies we reviewed is unknown, but would probably affect the data in both directions.

Despite our best efforts to reduce the amount of error in the estimates of response accuracy through a careful evaluation of the criteria applied and through some secondary data analysis, some error probably remains. We do not believe, however, that the amount of this error is significant in terms of its effect on our findings and conclusions.

We attribute our confidence in the data presented to several factors. First, each report was carefully scrutinized, with questions and data selected according to our stringent criteria. Second, we believe that we can be reasonably confident that the primary researchers exercised care and diligence in their data collection and analysis. Finally, our analysis does not depend on a single estimate of accuracy, but rather on percentages of accuracy estimated for approximately 250 questions.

Studies excluded are those in which informants were used as sources of response verification, such as in alcohol use and delinquency research, since the ultimate source of the informant's information may be the respondent, in which case reliability rather than validity is being assessed. Victimization studies were not included because in many cases the source of the police report with which the victimization report is compared is, again, the respondent.

Also excluded are studies where the criterion used for verification of responses is not directly tied to the behavior being measured, for example, liquor purchases and drinking. Although some researchers have used purchases to validate drinking reports, purchased liquor may not necessarily be consumed by the buyer or consumed within the specific time frame used in the question.

Finally, because we were only interested in studies in which the accuracy of individuals' responses was assessed, we excluded studies that reported findings in a form other than percentages of accurate responses and where the data could not be converted to percentages. For example, in some cases, results were reported in the form of a correlation, and response validity was not evaluated at the individual level. Although correlational data provides one type of assessment of the accuracy of survey responses, data reported in this form was not usable in this analysis.

Sixth, with respect to our meta-analysis, the studies were a source of speculation and hypotheses with respect to the identification of variables impacting accuracy levels. Our analysis, however, was theory driven as well, in that our selection of variables for analysis was guided by the literature in cognitive psychology and survey research.

The content of the studies reviewed varied greatly, for example, in the amount of detail reported, the frame of reference of the researchers, the goals and hypotheses of the researchers, and the overall quality of the analysis. Identifying the variables that might generally affect accuracy across the many types of studies required attempting to abstract the essential features of many of the questions and studies, often without knowing what the actual question posed to respondents had been. The variables we created for inclusion in the meta-analysis were largely the result of our interpretation of the reported information and often involved teasing out the relevant information where details were lacking or not obtainable. The actual impact on accuracy of these variables, and their relative power in terms of their association with accuracy, was then evaluated in a quantitative assessment.

Data Collection Procedures

An extensive search was conducted to identify appropriate studies for this investigation. *Psychological Abstracts*, as well as articles and books thought to have, or recommended as having, possible relevance were reviewed. All potentially pertinent references cited in any of the sources were thoroughly investigated.

In all, 37 studies were located which met our criteria and could therefore be included in this report. The publication dates for the reports of these studies ranged from 1944 to 1988. Many more studies were examined but did not lend themselves to the type of evaluation conducted herein. In all, the validity of responses made by 56,701 respondents to 258 questions was evaluated. These questions were grouped into topic areas.

Considering the vast number of research reports that have been published in the area of survey research, 37 reports may seem like a very small number. These studies were located, however, through a thorough and painstaking search. To the best of our knowledge, these studies represent the entire set of studies within the time frame of our search that fit within the framework of the criteria set forth in this report. It appears that in only a comparatively small number of studies have researchers attempted, using independent criteria, to assess the accuracy of individuals' responses to survey questions concerning behavior and personal characteristics. The unique analysis undertaken in this investigation could only have been conducted with questions from studies of this type.

The amount of detail with which information was reported in the studies varied widely. For example, in certain cases raw data were provided or extensive tables displayed, with full explanations of any data analyses performed. In other instances, only general conclusions were related. Differences in the way information is presented in this report reflect these variations.

Organization of This Book

Part II of this book is a general discussion of the studies included in this report. Each of the studies is presented in as much relevant detail as possible, including at a minimum a brief description of the study, a report of the percentages of accurate responding found for the particular questions included in the study, a discussion of the possible strengths and weaknesses of the study, a consideration of possible problems with the criteria used to validate responses, and the identification of factors potentially affecting response accuracy in that study.

The studies are categorized according to the general subjects of the questions. Question topic is widely believed to affect response accuracy. Organization by topic facilitates comparisons across questions concerning similar matters and, in doing so, permits a consideration of other factors that may account for differences in levels of response accuracy.

Chapter 3 focuses on comparatively nonthreatening topics, Chapter 4 includes sensitive topics, and Chapter 5 involves reports of financial matters. Accompanying tables summarize the studies according to specific topic headings. General findings and conclusions emerging from the analysis of the studies in Part II are discussed and summarized in Chapter 6.

In Part III, using data from the studies discussed in Part II, certain other issues in survey research are briefly explored. In Chapter 7, we investigate the aggregate level validity of survey data by means of comparisons of self-report with actual data. As in Part II, data is presented in tabular as well as narrative form. A second issue addressed in Chapter 7 is whether inaccurate reporting is item specific or a more general behavior associated with certain respondents. A chapter summary presents our conclusions with respect to these issues.

The meta-analysis of our data is reported in Part IV. Actually, three separate meta-analyses were performed. In Chapter 8, we describe the process of the selection of variables for inclusion in the meta-analysis, as well as our procedures for measuring or coding these variables. The rationale for the formation of data subsets is also presented. Results of the three analyses are described and discussed in Chapter 9. In Chapter 10, we attempt to integrate the results of the analyses and to identify common factors. An overall summary of our findings, along with our conclusions, is presented in Chapter 11.

In Part V, Chapter 12 contains a general summary of this investigation.

Part II

Accuracy Levels in Surveys: Factors Affecting Response Accuracy

2

Accuracy Levels in Surveys: Factors Affecting Response Accuracy — Introduction

In the following three chapters, the questions from the research reports included in this exploration are described and analyzed. The rationale for providing this detailed review was presented in Chapter 1. Briefly, secondary analysis of data presented in the original research reports was often required. Discussions in the review of the research will explain any apparent discrepancies and clarify our approach to the data.

Further, the detailed discussion of the studies allows the reader to follow us in our attempt to identify the relevant details or features of the surveys and questions which appeared to contribute to or detract from response accuracy. In this attempt, we were aided by the speculations occasionally offered by the primary authors. Being closest to the data and the data-gathering enterprise, the insights of these researchers are important to consider. For the most part, however, the goals of the primary researchers did not include a focus on the variables affecting accuracy. More frequently, then, the interpretations and observations offered in this regard are our own.

As we started our exploration, we were guided by the efforts of previous researchers to identify factors associated with response error. Lansing, Ginsburg, & Braaten (1961), Cannell & Kahn (1968), and Mauldin & Marks (1950), for example, identified three general classes of reasons for response error. These were:

1. *Inaccessibility of the information to the respondent.* A respondent simply may not have the requested information or be unable to remember it, particularly if the recall period is long and if the behavior or event in ques-

tion was not significant to the respondent. Over time, distortions of what is recalled are also possible. Further, records may not be available for consultation.

2. *Problems of communication.* If the specific question lacks clarity, is complex, or is set within a context that creates ambiguity, the respondent may not understand what information is being requested. Respondents may also misinterpret a question, attaching their own meaning to it, based, perhaps, on their perceptions of the survey's purposes or the interviewer's expectations. It is likely that respondents do not wish to appear uninformed, uncooperative, or unable to supply the information. Therefore, responses will probably be provided without requests for clarification.

3. *Motivational factors.* For various reasons, perhaps due to the sensitivity of the subject, the respondent may not be willing to supply accurate information and may deliberately conceal or distort the facts.

The suggestions of these and other researchers were useful in considering and organizing the factors believed to have affected the accuracy of respondents' replies in the following discussion of the studies. Our approach to the data, however, was not constrained by previous efforts. Rather, we turned to the data as our major source of information. Many of the factors that we believed were important to consider emerged during the course of our investigation.

Although we identified a large number of potentially influential variables, we found that information on many of these factors was not available across all of the studies. For example, information on the question context or on whether or not categories were used was often not presented. Our goal was to integrate the material and place the questions into a standardized framework in order to quantitatively and systematically assess the factors affecting accuracy. Toward this end, we sought to identify factors that could be emphasized across all of the studies. At the same time, we sought to explore as many of the potentially important variables as possible.

After we had identified certain key variables for analysis, we explored research and theories in other disciplines as they related to survey response accuracy. Our goal was to include in our meta-analysis not only those variables that emerged from the data, but to also explore factors suggested by theory and research in other potentially relevant areas. In other words, although we looked to the studies as a major source of hypotheses about the factors influencing accuracy, we were guided in our selection of variables for our meta-analysis by relevant theories and research in disciplines other than survey research. The process of the selection of variables for the meta-analysis is discussed fully in Chapter 8.

Because the subject of a survey question may influence respondents' truthfulness, and to facilitate comparisons, questions from the studies included in this discussion are organized according to topic. Questions on topics considered comparatively nonthreatening are examined first in Chapter 3, followed in Chapter 4 by a discussion of questions on sensitive subjects. Questions about financial matters, including tax-paying behavior questions, are discussed separately in Chapter 5.

For easy reference, each of the studies discussed is also briefly summarized in one of the tables accompanying these chapters. These summaries include a description of the sample, the method used, the response rate, the question(s) asked, the number of persons asked, the criterion against which responses were compared, the percentage of accurate responses, and the percentages of over- and underestimates. As previously mentioned, presenting the information in this standardized form frequently necessitated a considerable amount of reworking and reanalyzing of the data obtained from the original research reports.

As used in this report, the terms *overreporting* and *overclaiming* usually refer to instances when subjects falsely claim that they performed or possess something or that an event occurred, or when they report more than the correct amount. *Underreports* and *underclaims* are false reports in the other direction, such as denials or failures to admit acts that were actually performed.

It is also important to consider whether the sample included only owners or those known to have performed the behavior in question. The percentages of accurate responses for reverse record check samples[1] may not be comparable to the percentages for general samples because there is a greater effect on error with reverse record check samples. If the topic being discussed is considered sensitive, private, or socially undesirable, the amount of error is probably overstated (Horvitz, 1974; Ferber, Forsythe, Guthrie, & Maynes, 1969a,b); if the behavior is socially approved, the amount of error will tend to be understated unless the population of concern is owners or performers only.

For example, assume that 10% of the general population received public assistance income in 1959 and that the rate of denial among a sample of recipients is 7%. Also assume that nonrecipients rarely falsely claim having received benefits and are, therefore, 99% accurate. The error rate for a general sample would then be reduced to less than 2%.

---

[1]The term *reverse record check sample* as used in this report refers to cases where all of the respondents were involved in the subject in question. In most of these cases, the original sample consisted of these owners or performers. However, in certain other cases, the validation data provided referred only to those involved in the behavior.

As an example of a socially approved behavior, consider voting. In a sample of voters only, it is likely that a very high percentage of the respondents would truthfully report having voted. With a general sample, however, a sizable proportion of nonvoters can be expected to falsely claim that they voted, thereby increasing the overall amount of error.

For some types of questions, the probable effect on error of using a reverse record check rather than a general sample is less clear. For example, consider questions concerning savings account ownership. Many account owners may think of the matter as private and deny ownership. On the other hand, non-owners may feel that having an account is socially desirable and, therefore, falsely claim ownership.

Percentage of accuracy figures may also not be directly comparable be-tween studies due to differences in the standards for accuracy used. For example, in studies of amounts in savings accounts, some researchers counted a response as correct only if it was to the exact dollar, others if it was within a specific range, and others if it was within a given percentage of the true amount.

3

Reports on Comparatively Nonthreatening Topics

Reports of Descriptive Information

Three different research efforts were identified in this area. In a study reported by Cahalan (1968)[1], Denver residents were questioned face-to-face about their age, possession of a driver's license and library card, automobile and home ownership, and whether they had a telephone in the household. Accuracy was quite high, ranging from 83 to 98% (see Table 3.1).

Respondents' age reports were checked against both driver's license records and election registration records, with the driver's license comparisons yielding a higher percentage of agreement (92 versus 83%). Parry & Crossley (1950) offered several possible explanations:

> ... that the registration records are less accurate than the license records, that some respondents are *motivated to give less valid reports to registration officers*[2], or that the people for whom the various checks were possible *differ in their tendencies to give invalid answers to the official reporters and to interviewers.* [p. 79, emphases added]

Since only males were included in the election registration records check, possible sex differences in accuracy must be considered.

Cahalan argued that responses may be highly accurate to issues of present reality, such as those issues represented by all of the above questions, because

---

[1]Different aspects of this study, relevant to this exploration, were reported in the three studies listed in Table 3.1.

[2]However, these age questions were included in this report as it was assumed that some proof of age was required both to obtain a driver's license and to register to vote.

Table 3.1 Accuracy of Reports of Descriptive Information

Study	Sample description	Method	Response rate (%)	Information requested	Number asked	Criterion	Accurate responses %	Over/under (%)
Cahalan (1968); Parry & Crossley (1950); Crossley & Fink (1951)	1949 Area probability sample of 1349 names from the Denver city directory	Face to face	68.3 (N = 920)	Possession of driver's license	920	Official records	88	10/2
				Possession of a valid library card	902[a]	Official records	88.7	9.2/2
				Automobile ownership	892[b]	Official records	97	3/0[c]
				Home ownership	920[a]	Official records	96	3/1
				Telephone in household	920[e]	Official records	98	1/1
				Age	411[f]	Driver's license records	92[g]	4/4
				Age	297[k]	Election registration records	83[l]	8/9
Weaver & Swanson (1974)	Random sample of 600 male employees of the San Antonio fire and police departments	Telephone	56.6 (N = 339)	Date of birth	321[l]	Records of the City of San Antonio personnel office	91.8[k]	4.1/4.1
				Date employment began	313[l]	Records of the City of San Antonio personnel office	63.6[m]	20.1/16.3

Locander et al. (1976)	Probability sample of 464 Chicago households with telephones	Face to face	76.0 (N = 95)	Possession of library card	93"	Chicago Public Library records	81	19/0
		Telephone	89.9 (N = 98)	Possession of library card	97	Chicago Public Library records	79	21/0
		Questionnaire	75.4 (N = 86)	Possession of library card	82	Chicago Public Library records	82	18/0
		Random response	77.6 (N = 90)	Possession of library card	61	Chicago Public Library records	74[o]	26/0

[a]Excludes 18 "don't remember" or "no answer" responses = (2%).

[b]Excludes 28 "don't remember" or "no answer" responses = (3%).

[c]All "do not own" responses were assumed to be correct and not checked against records.

[d]Parry & Crossley (1950) report an N of 919 for this question.

[e]Parry & Crossley (1950) report an N of 918 for this question.

[f]Includes only those who had a driver's license.

[g]Within 1 year.

[h]Includes only male registrants.

[i]Within 1 year.

[j]Excludes 18 refusals = (5%).

[k]Within less than 1 year.

[l]Excludes 26 refusals = (8%).

[m]Within 30 days.

[n]The numbers differ from the overall number of actual respondents for each method due to some nonresponse to this particular question. Also, for the random response method "the sample size is estimated as 70 percent of those responding, since the remaining 30 percent answered a different question" (Locander et al., 1976, p. 271).

[o]For the random response method "the proportion of incorrect responses is estimated as the difference between the total population estimate using validation data and the estimate obtained from using ... [a measure of the sample estimate]. It is, of course, impossible to specify which respondents have given incorrect responses" (Locander et al., 1976, p. 271).

they present less strain on the respondent's memory than questions concerning past behavior. The operation of status enhancement or self-presentation factors may account for the greater number of overreports than underreports on questions about the possession of a driver's license or valid library card and about automobile or home ownership. Inaccurate responses to questions concerning age were divided about equally between overstatements and understatements.

Using the telephone rather than the face-to-face interview method, Weaver & Swanson (1974), in their study of San Antonio fire and police department employees, also found a high percentage (91.8%) of accurate responses to an age question and an equal distribution of inaccurate reports between overstatements and understatements (see Table 3.1). In this study, respondents were asked about their date of birth rather than their age.[3]

On the question concerning when the respondents started working at their jobs, which the authors called job seniority, the percentage of accurate responses fell to 63.6%, with the number of overstatements being somewhat greater than the number of understatements. A response was considered accurate if it was within 30 days of the criterion date. Job seniority is not likely as salient a fact as date of birth; some thought is required to recall the date that employment began.

It is also possible that the question lacked clarity. The exact question asked was "When did you start working there?" (p. 71). Yet in discussing the inaccuracy, the authors stated that it was well known among employees that the accumulation of seniority begins at the end of a 6-month probationary period. Apparently the probationary period was a training period. Whether the actual question was interpreted by the respondents as referring to the date seniority began or the date the training program began cannot be known. Yet the consistent reference to seniority suggests that the seniority date was the criterion used by the authors.

Locander *et al.* (1976) examined the effects of method on the validity of responses to several questions put to Chicago household members, including one question concerning the possession of a library card (see Table 3.1). The percentages of accurate responses were at a moderate level and were similar for the face-to-face interview (81%), telephone (79%), and questionnaire methods (82%). The random response method had the lowest percentage of accurate responses (74%), but this is an estimate.[4] However, an analysis of the

---

[3]Again, it was assumed that some proof of age was required for employment in either the fire or the police departments.

[4]Since it is not possible to assess the accuracy of an individual's response in the random response method condition, no other studies using this method are reported. However, the results are included in this case since the authors analyzed the data over all methods used.

data by the authors over all questions and methods in the study revealed no significant method effect. The operation of self-presentation or social desirability influences are again likely because, for all methods, inaccurate responses were exclusively overstatements.

Why the subjects in Cahalan's (1968) study were somewhat more accurate concerning the possession of a library card than were the respondents interviewed face-to-face in Locander *et al.*'s study (88.7 versus 81%) is not evident, although sample differences may have been a factor.

Reports of Various Events and Behaviors

Three studies on a variety of subjects were grouped to facilitate discussion. Weiss (1968) checked the responses of black welfare mothers to two questions about their children: had they failed a subject on their last report cards, and had they ever been required to repeat a grade in school. The percentage of accurate responses to the subject failure question was low (63%), with most of the inaccuracy consisting of understatements (27%) (see Table 3.2). The higher percentage of accurate responses to the grade failure question (78%) may be because grade failure is not common. A truthful "no" response, therefore, is highly probable.

The number of overstatements to these questions is somewhat puzzling. Weiss explained this outcome, which she termed "reverse error, or confusion" (p. 623), with the suggestion that "many mothers were *unaware* of the facts on children's school performance" (p. 623, emphasis added).

Hyman (1944) used a direct mailing list for government posters to sample and survey storekeepers about receipt of these posters in general, and receipt of the most recent one, mailed about 10 days prior to the survey. These posters were probably war effort posters, given the study date of 1944.

Eighty-six percent of the respondents stated that they had received posters, but only 32.5% of these said they had received the most recent poster (see Table 3.2). These 221 storekeepers were then asked if they had the poster on display. If they said yes, the interviewer asked to see the displayed poster. Forty-six percent of the respondents who said they had received the poster also said it was on display, but only 4% of the group actually had it on display.

Hyman was confident that the storekeepers had actually received the recent poster, because a check in each sample district revealed that at least some grocers had received it. However, it is possible that many of the storekeepers did not take responsibility for receiving the mail, or perhaps, as Hyman suggested, tended to forget or ignore mailings of this sort.

Table 3.2 Accuracy of Reports of Various Events and Behaviors

Study	Sample description	Method	Response rate (%)	Information requested	Number asked	Criterion	Accurate responses %	Over/under (%)
Weiss (1968)	Black welfare mothers residing in New York City who received public assistance in 1966 and who had been interviewed by the National Opinion Research Center for a study on the use of health services[c]	Face to face	NA[a] (N = 1002)	Child's failure of a subject on his last report card	416[b]	Official records	63	10/27
				Child's ever being left back to repeat a grade in school	400	Official records	78	12/10
Hyman (1944)	Grocery stores on a direct mailing list to receive government posters	Face to face	NA (N = 790)	Whether received government posters	790	Direct mailing list	86	−[a]/14
				Whether received a specific poster known to have been mailed about 10 days earlier	679	Direct mailing list	32.5	−/67.5
				Whether poster was put on display	221	Display check	58	42/0[a]

Clancy, et al., (1979)	National probability sample of approximately 1000 subscribers to a magazine appealing to middle- and upper-income households	Face to face	NA[a] (N = 1053)	Whether they had read in the current issue any of four full-length articles, four brief articles, or four advertisements which were actually scheduled to run in future issues of the magazine	514[f]	Actual current contents of the magazine	36.5 (full-length articles)	63.5/—
							44.7 (short articles)	55.3/—
							24.2 (advertise-ments)	75.8/—

[a] For this and all tables herein, NA = not available.

[b] The author reports that "the number of cases for which school data could be checked was reduced because families had no child in New York City public schools at the fourth grade level or above, because records were lost or unavailable in the schools, because children could not be located in the schools reported, and not every school could be visited before the end of the school year" (Weiss, 1968, p. 623).

[c] Actually, a small number of respondents were no longer receiving welfare assistance by the time the interviews were conducted.

[d] For this and all tables herein, signifies situation arising in a reverse record check study whereby this type of response was not possible.

[e] Respondents' reports that the poster was *not* on display were not checked.

[f] The authors report that approximately 50% (N = 514) of the original sample reported looking at, or reading, a current issue of the magazine. The relevant information was then requested of these respondents.

Nevertheless, the high rate of inaccurate responses to the question concerning the display of the posters is interesting. Distortion was apparently all in the direction of overstatement. ("No" responses to this question were not checked.) This again suggests a self-presentation or social desirability effect, since the display of what were likely wartime posters would be indicative of patriotic sentiments.

In an investigation of the accuracy of self-reports of magazine readership by subscribers, Clancy, Ostlund, & Wyner (1979) found that about 76% of the respondents claimed to have read at least one advertisement, 55% at least one brief article, and 64% at least one full-length article, all of which had actually not yet been published (see Table 3.2).

The authors investigated a possible social desirability effect — measured by assessing the respondent's need for social approval and trait desirability or attitude toward the magazine — and concluded that only a partial explanation for the high percentages of overstatements was provided. They suggested the investigation of other factors, such as acquiescence response set (meaning the tendency to agree with survey items regardless of content) and interest in the subject matter.

These low levels of response accuracy are partially explained by the fact that, for each question, the subjects were actually presented with four items, namely, four advertisements, brief articles, or full-length articles. A response was then made concerning the readership of each item. As more items were presented, more respondents provided false claims.

Reports of Attendance and Absenteeism

Hyman (1944), using two methods and samples, queried workers in two industrial plants concerning absences from work. In each plant, a group of workers who had been absent most recently was surveyed about their recent absences by means of what Hyman (1944) referred to as an "intensive" (p. 558) face-to-face interview. These groups had over 96% accuracy, with all distortions being understatements (see Table 3.3). The other sample, a cross-section of workers in the two plants, received a questionnaire. Only 66.4% of those respondents who had been absent reported truthfully regarding their absences in the last two months, while 33.6% failed to report recorded absences.

Hyman suggested that the lower rate of accuracy in the second sample may be attributed to errors of recall because these workers' absences were not all as recent as the absences for the first sample. The 2-month time frame used, however, is still relatively short.

Table 3.3 Accuracy of Reports of Attendance and Absenteeism

Study	Sample description	Method	Response rate (%)	Information requested	Number asked	Criterion	Accurate responses %	Over/under (%)
Hyman (1944)	Workers in two industrial plants who had all been absent recently[a]	Face to face	NA (N = 158)	Whether absent recently	158	Plant records	96.2	−/3.8
	Cross-section of workers in two industrial plants	Questionnaire	NA (N = 200)	Whether absent in the last couple of months	134[b]	Plant records	66.4	−/33.6
Gray (1955)	Employees present in a group of British government offices during a period of about 2 hours on the morning of November 15	Questionnaire	NA[c]	Whether sick leave taken in the period July–Nov. 15	433	Employer's sick leave records	91.5[d]	3.0/5.5
Hagburg (1968)	Local union leaders participating in a long-term union leadership program conducted by the Ohio State University	Questionnaire	NA (N = 227)	How many union leadership program classes attended the first 8 weeks of this year	227	Official attendance records	53	41/6
				How many union leadership program classes attended the second 8 weeks of this year	227	Official attendance records	48	38/15

[a]The same two industrial plants were used as in the following study, and the two surveys were conducted simultaneously.

[b]Represents the number of respondents who "had records of recent absences" (Hyman, 1944, p. 558).

[c]Some questionnaire forms were discarded in cases where it was believed that respondents had learned of the inquiry in advance and may have had an opportunity to consult records. A few more were not used due to some confusion in the employer's records or where the questionnaires were incomplete. The exact number of these discarded and unused forms was not given.

[d]Represents those who admitted or correctly denied having taken at least some sick leave in the survey period.

All distortion was in the direction of understatements. Workers may be reluctant to admit absenteeism because absences are incongruent with the image of a good worker or because they perceive absences to be socially undesirable. Perhaps these considerations aren't as important for the first sample of workers, who had all recently been absent and who may also tend to be absent frequently. The possible effect of method — intensive face-to-face interview versus questionnaire — must also be considered.

Gray (1955) was interested in determining if British government employees could recall not only the amount of sick leave they had taken, but also when it had been taken. Over 91% of the respondents either correctly denied or admitted taking sick leave during the 4½-month period immediately preceding the survey (see Table 3.3)[5]. However, of the 228 persons who had taken at least some sick leave, only 74 were completely accurate, 24 recorded no leave, 22 noted the correct month but the wrong amount, and 108 gave correct amounts but wrong month responses. Of the 205 subjects who had not taken any sick leave, 13 reported doing so.

Gray attributed the inaccuracy to forgetting, and mainly to forgetting the time when the absences occurred. He reasoned that some error in providing estimates concerning behavior of this type, which is ongoing, is affected by experience outside of the particular reference period. For example, illness and resulting sick leave taken prior to the reference period may be incorrectly recalled as occurring during this period.

In Hagburg's (1968) study, when local union leaders were asked immediately following the second 8-week period about their attendance in a union leadership program, only 53% gave accurate responses concerning the first 8 weeks of the program. Accuracy dropped to 48% for the second 8 weeks, or more recent half of the program (see Table 3.3). The percentage of respondents who correctly reported their attendance for the 16 weeks of classes, or who answered both attendance questions accurately, was just 36%.

Hagburg concluded that the proximity of the event in time did not appear to have influenced the accuracy of respondents' reports for the two time periods. As might be predicted, inaccurate responses were overwhelmingly overstatements, and the number of these was fairly consistent over time. According to the report, all participants in these classes were told that attendance was encouraged and necessary to qualify for a certification of completion. Hagburg suggested that the responses tended to reflect these explicit expectations, or ideal norms.

---

[5]After being presented with a form on which the months in question were indicated, employees were asked to note the number of sick days taken in each month.

Reports of Hospitalization Episodes

Cannell & Fowler (1963) were interested not only in ascertaining the accuracy of survey data, but also the relative accuracy of the face-to-face interview and questionnaire techniques in the reporting of information about hospitalizations. In this study, the questionnaires were left with the respondent to be returned by mail.

The percentages of accuracy for this study are the percentages of episodes correctly reported rather than the percentages of truthful respondents as in previous studies. The number of respondents, however, is fairly similar to the number of episodes for both procedures, the ratios being 462:521 for the face-to-face interview and 465:546 for the questionnaire. The reporting period was 1 year prior to the interview. Proxy respondents, or other household members, were used for children under 18 or for respondents who were not at home.

The authors concluded that, in general, the results from the two procedures were similar (see Table 3.4). The question concerning whether surgery was performed produced the highest percentage of accurate responses for both the face-to-face interview and the questionnaire (90 and 91%, respectively). Inaccurate reports were exclusively understatements. For the total number of hospitalizations question, both techniques also had similar results (83 versus 84%); all distortions were again underreports.

Respondents in the questionnaire procedure were reportedly significantly more accurate on the length of stay question (57 versus 42% correct) and somewhat more accurate concerning the month of discharge (83 versus 77% correct) than respondents who were interviewed face to face.[6] The authors suggested that this information is most likely available in records, and respondents in the questionnaire procedure were able to check records or consult with other people. However, response accuracy to the length of stay question was low for both groups.

On the other hand, those interviewed face to face were slightly more accurate concerning diagnosis (65 versus 61% correct) and type of surgery (75 versus 69% correct). The authors stated that records are least likely to be available for this type of information, but interviewers can motivate the respondents to obtain a full report.

For these two questions, when findings from both methods were compared with respect to the reporting of what were labeled "embarrassing . . .

---

[6]Variances were estimated "using the formula 1.5 (pq/n), which we have found to provide a conservative estimate of variance. Using this basis, we state that a difference is 'significant' when it exceeds two standard errors, $p<.05$" (Cannell & Fowler, 1963, p. 255).

Table 3.4 Accuracy of Reports of Hospitalization Episodes

Study	Sample description	Method	Response rate (%)	Information requested	Number asked	Criterion	Accurate responses %	Over/under (%)
Cannell & Fowler (1963)	Individuals selected on a probability basis from a probability sample of general hospitals in the Detroit area, stratified by hospital size. All individuals had one or more discharges during the sample period (May, 1960–March, 1961), after hospitalization for one or more nights' duration (excluding normal deliveries).	Face to face	96[a]	Total number of hospital episodes	462	Hospital records	83[b]	0/17
				Length of hospital stay	NA[c]	Hospital records	42[d]	NA/NA
				Month of discharge	NA	Hospital records	77	NA/NA
				Diagnosis	NA	Hospital records	65	NA/NA
				Whether surgery was performed	NA	Hospital records	90	0/10
				Type of surgery, if any	NA	Hospital records	75	NA/NA
		Questionnaire[e]	92	Total number of hospital episodes	465	Hospital records	84	0/16
				Length of hospital stay	NA[f]	Hospital records	57	NA/NA
				Month of discharge	NA	Hospital records	83	NA/NA
				Diagnosis	NA	Hospital records	61	NA/NA
				Whether surgery was performed	NA	Hospital records	91	0/9
				Type of surgery, if any	NA	Hospital records	69	NA/NA

[a] For both methods, the authors report that some of these cases were deleted, after editing. However, they do not indicate the exact number of these.

[b] Indicates the percentage of "episodes" reported correctly. There were 521 "episodes" connected with the 462 respondents in the interview procedure, and 546 "episodes" connected with the 465 respondents in the self-administered questionnaire method condition.

[c] Approximately 83% of the 521 episodes, or 431 episodes, were reported. The number of respondents associated with these 431 episodes is not given.

[d] For this and the following four questions, for both methods, refers to the percentage of episodes for which the information was correct.

[e] However, for this sample, the data concerning visits to doctors, chronic and acute conditions, and demographic status were collected by means of a personal interview. Also, if respondents failed to return the questionnaire within a specified period of time, a second form was sent. If this form was not returned, respondents were interviewed by telephone where possible (13% of the sample) or in person (3% of the sample).

[f] Approximately 84% of the 546 episodes, or 459 episodes, were reported. The number of respondents associated with these 459 episodes is not given.

[or] ... threatening" (Cannell & Fowler, 1963, p. 256) diagnoses, no differences were found. The reporting of episodes involving "embarrassing" (p. 256) surgery, however, was better for the face-to-face interview technique than for the questionnaire procedure. The authors had predicted that the questionnaire procedure would be superior in this regard because of its greater impersonality. They surmised that their hypothesis was not confirmed because the respondents were not anonymous in this study.

That the questions on whether surgery was performed and on the total number of hospitalizations produced high percentages of accurate responses is not surprising, due to the salience of events of this type. It is also probable that many respondents did not know their diagnosis, which would account for the high inaccuracy rate for that question. The lowest percentage of accurate responses for both methods were concerning the length of hospital stay. It would have been interesting to know the degree of inaccuracy of responses to this question because it seems likely that, although it might be difficult to remember the exact number of days, estimates would be good approximations. Response error on this question might also have been high due to the length of the recall period and the consequent tax on the respondent's memory, especially in the face-to-face interview condition.

Concerning the use of proxy respondents, persons who answered for themselves in the face-to-face interview reportedly provided significantly[7] more accurate reports on the total number of hospitalizations question than proxy respondents for adults (13 versus 27% of episodes not reported). Proxy respondents for children were the most accurate for both methods. For the questionnaire method, however, the relationship of the respondent to the sample person made little difference in reporting accuracy overall. Reporting by proxy respondents for adults was more accurate than in the face-to-face interview condition (17 versus 27% of episodes not reported). The authors attributed these results to the ability of proxies to consult with family members while completing the questionnaire.

Concerning the question on the length of hospital stay, in both the questionnaire and the face-to-face interview procedures, proxy respondents' reports were again most accurate when the questions concerned their children. The questionnaire method produced the most accurate results for this question, especially when the respondent was a proxy for an adult (54 versus 29% of episodes correctly reported).

The authors also examined the effect on response error of the way in which follow-up was obtained. How the subjects responded to the data-collection efforts was viewed as a measure of their motivation. For those

---

[7]See footnote 6 in this chapter.

respondents who did not return the questionnaire within a specified period of time, a second questionnaire was provided. If the second questionnaire was not returned, respondents were contacted by telephone or in person. Those who returned either the first or the second forms were more accurate concerning the total number of hospitalizations than those contacted by telephone or in person (13 versus 15 versus 32% of episodes not reported). For the length of stay question, findings were similar (60 versus 53 versus 33% correctly reported). The researchers cautioned, however, that this difference may be attributable to procedure differences rather than to the level of motivation.

The authors suggested several conclusions based on their data. First, the effects on accurate reporting of certain factors, such as the use of proxy respondents, may differ depending on the method used. Second, the method—questionnaire versus face-to-face interview—that will produce the more accurate data depends on the type of information being requested. Third, anonymity may be a more important factor than the presence or absence of an interviewer in obtaining accurate reports concerning threatening questions.

Finally, their finding that reports obtained through follow-up efforts are progressively less accurate than the surveys completed on the first attempt suggests that respondents' motivation to participate may affect response accuracy.

Reports of Cigarette Smoking

When a sample of adolescents was questioned about the recency of their cigarette smoking, all gave accurate responses, whether or not they had been forewarned that a breath sample would be taken to validate their answers (see Table 3.5). This finding, in a study by Bauman, Koch, & Bryan (1982), was based on a comparison of self-reports with breath carbon monoxide concentrations, using a concentration level somewhat lower than that often used for adults to distinguish recent from nonrecent smokers. The authors stated that the exact level that should be used had still not been determined.

Reports of Voting Behavior

In a postelection voting survey for the 1964 presidential election, Clausen (1968) found that over 97% of the 1110 respondents for whom validating information was available were truthful in their responses (see Table 3.6). One possible explanation for this high degree of accuracy is that the survey also included a pre-election interview. Clausen stated that this may have

Table 3.5 Accuracy of Reports of Cigarette Smoking

Study	Sample description	Method	Response rate (%)	Information requested	Number asked	Criterion	Accurate responses %	Over/under (%)
Bauman, Koch, & Bryan (1982)	226 ninth graders enrolled in one junior high school in the Chapel Hill-Carrboro (North Carolina) City Schools. Assignment to Group I or II was random.	Questionnaire	36[a] (N = 82)					
		Group I – Respondents told that air sample would be taken		Recency of smoking cigarettes	43	Expired air carbon monoxide concentrations	100[b]	0/0
		Group II Respondents not informed that an air sample would be taken		Recency of smoking cigarettes	39	Expired air carbon monoxide concentrations	100	0/0

[a] Parental consent was obtained for 99 pupils. Of these, "one refused to provide an air specimen, and the rest either were inadvertently not contacted to participate in the study, or were absent during the day that data were collected, or no longer attended the school" (Bauman et at., 1982, 1132).
[b] Using 6 ppm as the cutoff, for both groups.

Table 3.6 Accuracy of Reports of Voting Behavior

Study	Sample description	Method	Response rate (%)	Information requested	Number asked	Criterion	Accurate responses %	Over/under (%)
Clausen (1968)	1565 pre-election respondents from a probability sample of 1932 eligible American voters residing in the 48 contiguous states and also residing in "distinctly indentifiable dwelling units commonly characterized by the possession of both dining and sleeping facilities that are not shared by the occupants of different dwelling units" (p. 591).	Face to face	92.3 (N = 1450)	Whether voted for president on Nov. 3, 1964	1110[a]	Official records	97.2	2.3/.5
Freeman (1953)	Residents of the state of Washington who were respondents in a pre-election survey	Face to face	84.8 (N = 374)[c]	Whether voted in recent (1950) election	374	Voting registration lists	82.6	15.2[b]/2.2
Miller (1952)	225 Pre-election respondents from a one-third probability sample (265 cases) of the adult population (age 21 and over) of the Precinct 13 in Waukegan, Illinois	Face to face	91.0 (N = 204)	Whether voted in recent (1950) congressional elections	204	County clerk's election registration and voting records	89.2	10.8/0

Study	Population	Method	Response rate (N)	Measure	N	Validation source	%	Ratio
Katosh & Traugott (1981)	National	Face to face	NA (N = 2304)	1978 Registration status	2230[i]	Official records	85.6	12.3/2.1
		Face to face	(N = 2415)	1978 Voting behavior	2222[k]	Official records	85.9	12.8/1.3
				1976 Registration status	2344[l]	Official records	84.6	12.3/3.2
			NA	1976 Voting behavior	2329[g]	Official records	86.5	12.3/1.2
Cahalan (1968); Parry & Crossley (1950); Crossley & Fink (1951)	See Table 3.1	Face to face	68.3 (N = 920)	Whether registered or voted in Denver 1943–1948[b]	920	Official records	82	16/2
				Whether voted in 1948 presidential election	920[c]	Official records	86	13/1
				Whether voted in Sept., 1948 primary election	856[f]	Official records	74.2	22.5/3.3
				Whether voted in 1947 City Charter election	828[e]	Official records	66.7	31.2/2.2
				Whether voted in May, 1947 mayoral election	911[i]	Official records	70.7	28.3/1
				Whether voted in Nov., 1946 congressional election	828[m]	Official records	76.7	21.1/2.2
				Whether voted in 1944 presidential election	902[n]	Official records	74.5	23.5/2
King et al. (1981)	Approximately 10% of the registered voters in a predominantly white, middle and working class residential community bordering Battle Creek, Michigan	Mailed questionnaire	51.4 (N = 215)	Whether voted in each of three recent school finance elections	215[o]	Voting registration rolls/voting records	32.1	51.2/4.7
Tittle & Hill (1967)	Students	Questionnaire	NA (N = 301)	Voting behavior in a student election 1 week prior	296[p]	Student voting records	90.5	9.5/0

(continues)

Table 3.6 (*continued*)

Study	Sample description	Method	Response rate (%)	Information requested	Number asked	Criterion	Accurate responses %	Over/under (%)
Locander *et al.* (1976)	See Table 3.1	Face to face	76.0 (N = 98)	Voter registration	93[a]	City voting records	85	15/0
		Telephone	89.9 (N = 98)	Voter registration	89	City voting records	83	17/0
		Questionnaire	75.4 (N = 86)	Voter registration	80	City voting records	88	12/0
		Random response	77.6 (N = 90)	Voter registration	61	City voting records	89[c]	11/0
		Face to face	76.0 (N = 95)	Whether voted in last (March, 1972, presidential) primary	80	City voting records	61	39/0
		Telephone	89.9 (N = 98)	Whether voted in last (March, 1972, presidential) primary	77	City voting records	69	31/0
		Questionnaire	75.4 (N = 86)	Whether voted in last (March, 1972, presidential) primary	74	City voting records	64	36/0
		Random response	77.6 (N = 90)	Whether voted in last (March, 1972, presidential) primary	50	City voting records	52[a]	48/0
Rogers (1976)	A reinterview of 247 residents in two New York City community planning districts, originally selected by quota and probability sampling methods, now stratified by ethnicity and	Method A: Telephone	NA[c]	Whether voted in the 1973 New York City mayoral election	81[a]	Voting records	79	20/1
		Method B: Face to face	NA	Whether voted in the 1973 New York City mayoral election	90	Voting records	71	26/4

age. All those without telephones or who did not speak English were excluded. Assignment to Method A or B was random.

[a] Represents the number of respondents for whom validating information was available.

[b] The authors caution that there may be some problems with the record check, such as individuals voting under different names (e.g., single names) than they used with the interviewer (e.g., married names).

[c] The authors initially report that 364 persons were interviewed. However, in the data presentation, the N reported is 374.

[d] Excludes 74 cases (3% of respondent total) where data were missing, records could not be checked, etc. Actually, in the 1978 study, and presumably in the 1976 study as well, the voting question was a filter for the registration question, with all "no" or "don't know" responses to the voting question being followed by the registration question. Therefore, the N's for the registration questions should be smaller. Since the reported N's are somewhat higher for the registration questions, it is concluded that the authors assumed that the respondents who reported voting would also have reported registration.

[e] Excludes 82 cases (4% of respondent total) where data were missing, records could not be checked, etc.

[f] Excludes 71 cases (3% of respondent total) where data were missing, records could not be checked, etc.

[g] Excludes 86 cases (4% of respondent total) where data were missing, records could not be checked, etc.

[h] According to Parry & Crossley (1950), this was two separate questions, with "yes" or "don't know" responses to the registration question being followed by the voting question. However, in all reports, responses to both questions are combined.

[i] Actually, questions about voting in specific elections were asked only of those who reported being registered to vote in Denver at some time since 1943 and who also reported having voting in an election in Denver since 1943. Apparently, it was assumed that those who reported that they had not been registered would also have denied any voting, and that those who denied having voted since 1943 would have denied voting in any specific election.

[j] Excludes 64 "don't remember" or "no answer" responses (7%).

[k] Excludes 92 "don't remember" or "no answer" responses (10%).

[l] Excludes 9 "don't remember" or "no answer" responses (1%).

[m] Excludes 92 "don't remember" or "no answer" responses (10%).

[n] Excludes 18 "don't remember" or "no answer" responses (2%).

[o] Includes 26 cases, or 12.1% of the sample, where respondents reported not remembering whether they had voted.

[p] Excludes five respondents for whom validating data could not be found.

[q] The numbers asked differ from the overall number of actual respondents "because on the validation of voter registration and voting some of the records were in litigation and were not available" (Locander et al., 1976, p. 271). Also, see footnote " in Table 3.1.

[r] See footnote " in Table 3.1.

[s] See footnote " in Table 3.1.

[t] The overall response rate was 82%. However, the response rate by method was not given.

[u] At one point, the author reported that voting information was available for a total of 169 respondents. However, in a tabular presentation of data, the total N was 171.

stimulated the respondents to vote, and those who vote are highly unlikely to give inaccurate voting reports.

In fact, the turnout estimate for Clausen's group, based on the number of responses that were validated, was 75.1%, which is unusually high. In Weiss's (1968) presentation of data from five voting studies, the percentages of actual voters ranged from 47 to 61%. However, samples may differ in voting behavior irrespective of pre-election interview exposure. Unlike the samples in the studies cited by Weiss, Clausen's was a national sample.

Another influence on voting behavior may be the particular election, due to differences in candidates' popularity or issues. Presidential elections typically have higher turnouts. In fact, the highest turnout in the studies cited by Weiss occurred in a presidential election voting study.

Finally, although the survey dates are not mentioned in Clausen's report, it appears that the survey was conducted shortly after the election. The length of the recall period, then, was probably short.

In Freeman's (1953) analysis of the state of Washington's voting survey data, overall accuracy was about 83%, with most distortions being overstatements (see Table 3.6). Like Clausen (1968), Freeman's data was from postelection reinterviews reportedly conducted shortly after the election, but the overall level of accuracy was not as high as that found by Clausen (97.2%). The percentage of actual voters (58.3%), although substantial, was also lower than the percentage in Clausen's report (75.1%).

Freeman concluded that a sample of respondents who are willing to participate in reinterviews has a higher proportion of voters than the general population. Freeman's accuracy and actual voter figures were lower than Clausen's possibly because Clausen's data were for a presidential election, while Freeman's were for an off-year (1950) election. Sample differences must also be considered.

Miller (1952) also conducted pre- and postelection interviews concerning the 1950 off-year congressional elections in a predominantly Republican precinct in Waukegan, Illinois. The postelection survey was conducted within about a month following the election (see Table 3.6). A higher percentage of the responses was accurate (89.2%) than for Freeman's sample (82.6%), with all distortions being overreports. In this group, 53.9% of the respondents voted, which is slightly less than the percentage of voters in Freeman's sample (58.3%).

Katosh & Traugott (1981) specifically sought to compare data from the 1976 presidential election with data from the off-year election of 1978 to determine whether response accuracy varies with the particular electoral context. Both sets of data were from the Center for Political Studies' *National Election Studies*. These surveys started the day after the election and continued until late December.

In the 1978 study, and presumably in the 1976 study as well, only persons who reported not having voted or who responded "don't know," were asked about registration. For the 1978 study, respondents who reported being registered to vote were asked to provide their registration address. Approximately 11% of those claiming to be registered reported a registration address other than their current address. This extended inquiry permitted a more accurate response check.

Similar high percentages of accurate responses were obtained in 1976 and 1978 for both the registration (84.6 and 85.6%) and the voting questions (86.5 and 85.9%). Distortions were again mainly overreports (see Table 3.6). The validation check also showed that presidential election voter turnout rates, at least for 1976, were higher (60.8%) than those for the 1978 off-year election (43.2%).

A substantially lower rate of accuracy would be expected for the 1976 registration question because the validation procedure, as explained above, was less precise than in 1978. That this expectation was not met is partially attributable to the higher voter turnout in 1976 and the resultant decreased number of "no" or "don't know" responses to the voting question (683 versus 1054 in 1978). Assuming that the same percentage of respondents would have reported registration at other than their current address in both 1976 and 1978, just 15 responses were incorrectly classified in 1976, while in 1978, 45 answers were subject to the improved verification process.

The Denver Validity Study discussed above, conducted in April and May of 1949, included eight questions on registration and voting (see Table 3.6). Unlike most of the other surveys reported in this section, respondents were asked not only about recent electoral behavior, but also about registration and voting behavior within an approximate 6-year period. Over time, decline in accuracy due to errors in recall is expected. On the other hand, particular election characteristics may influence memory and reporting.

Looking at the percentages of "don't remember" or "no answer" responses to the six specific election questions reveals that more of those types of responses ("don't remembers," etc.) were given to questions about the 1947 city charter (10%), the 1946 congressional (10%), and the 1948 presidential primary (7%) elections than to questions about the 1944 presidential (2%) and the 1947 mayoral (1%) elections, elections which generated more voter interest (see Table 3.6). Concerning the most recent election, the 1948 presidential, none of the respondents failed to answer or reported not remembering.

The highest percentage (86%) of accurate responses to all of the specific election questions was for the most recent election, and the next highest percentages (76.7 and 74.5%, respectively) were for the most remote elections, the 1946 congressional and the 1944 presidential. The lowest percentage (66.7%) was for the 1947 city charter election. These data support the conclusion that some elections are more memorable than others, irrespective of their recency. For all voting questions, distortions were mainly overstatements.

Overall, response error was much greater on questions of past behavior than for the present status questions included in Cahalan's (1968) study (see Table 3.1). Cahalan suggested that individuals' responses to the voting questions may have been based more on their sense of what they should have done, and may have come to believe they did, than what actually occurred. The frequency with which an individual performs the behavior is another explanation for error. If individuals usually vote, they may be more likely to assume that they voted in any specific election, especially when the election in question occurred some years ago.

Cahalan also described other potential sources of error and factors that may have contributed to accuracy. For example, he noted that Parry & Crossley (1950) had discussed the fact that if the behavior in question had a high incidence of performance within the group being surveyed, and errors tended to be overreports, then responses in general were more likely to be accurate. In fact, we found a significant positive Pearson correlation ($r = .69$, $df = 10$, $p \leq .01$) between the percentages of accurate responses and the percentages of respondents who performed the behavior for all of the questions included in the Denver survey, except the questions on age, where performance did not apply, and the question on registration and voting, which actually was a combination of two queries (see Table 3.7). For all of these items, a "yes" response was apparently prestige or status enhancing. Errors were mostly overstatements.

One potential difficulty in interpreting Cahalan's findings involves the clarity of the questions asked, with implications for the classification of responses as accurate or inaccurate and for the determination of voter turnout rates. Respondents were initially asked if they had "been registered to vote in Denver at any time since 1943" (Parry & Crossley, 1950, p. 73). Those who responded "yes" or "don't know" were then asked whether they had "voted in any election in Denver since 1943" (Parry & Crossley, 1950, p. 73). Those who responded "yes" to that question were asked about voting in specific elections. The specific election questions, however, were not followed by the phrase "in Denver," and only Denver records were used to validate responses.

As an example of a possible problem, an individual may have recently moved to Denver and both registered and voted there. However, he or she may have voted elsewhere in the 1944 presidential election. His or her "yes" response to the 1944 presidential election question would have been classified as incorrect, although not untruthful.

Table 3.7   Comparison between Performance and Accurate Behavioral Reports for Cahalan's (1968) Items

Information requested	Percentage performing	Percentage correct reports
Telephone in household	85.0	98.0
Whether voted in 1948 presidential election	61.0	86.0
Automobile ownership	60.9	97.0
Home ownership	54.0	96.0
Possession of driver's license	46.0	88.0
Whether voted in 1944 presidential election	38.8	74.5
Whether voted in May, 1947 mayoral election	36.3	70.7
Whether voted in Nov., 1946 congressional election	32.2	76.7
Whether voted in Sept., 1948 primary election	29.0	74.2
Whether contributed or pledged money to Community Chest in Fall, 1948 drive	27.8	62.2
Whether voted in 1947 City Charter election	21.1	66.7
Valid library card	13.3	88.7

As another example, respondents may have correctly denied being registered or having voted in Denver, yet those individuals may have voted elsewhere in specific elections. The responses would have been considered accurate, but the calculation of election turnout rates for the sample of respondents would have been incorrect. Also, respondents underreporting registration would not have been asked the voting questions. Some may have voted but were not given the opportunity to affirm or deny it. Although only a few respondents appear to fall into this category, exactly how their nonresponses to voting questions were considered is not known.

King, Lewis, & Rogers (1981) checked the voting reports of a Michigan community's registered voters for each of three recent (within about 1 year) school finance elections, and found that only 32.1% of the sample correctly reported their voting behavior (see Table 3.6). More than one-half of the sample claimed to have voted in at least one election although records indicated otherwise. Typical of voting surveys, underreports were few. The results from King *et al.*'s study are not strictly comparable with the other studies because these data are concerned with truthfulness on three questions grouped together.

Tittle & Hill (1967) found that 90.5% of their student respondents told the truth when asked about participation in a student election held 1 week prior to the survey (see Table 3.6). The nature of the election, the sample, and the short time frame involved probably contributed to the high degree of accuracy.

In Locander *et al.*'s (1976) study of Chicago households, the effect of method was assessed for questions on voter registration and voting in the last primary election (see Table 3.6). Consistent with other studies cited, high percentages of accurate responses were obtained for the registration question for all methods: face-to-face interview (85%), telephone (83%), questionnaire (88%), and random response (89%).

In contrast, the question on voting in the last primary evoked large numbers of inaccurate responses with the percentages of correct responses ranging from 52 to 69%. One possible explanation is that this election took place at least 8 months prior to the survey. Another is that primary elections probably have low turnout rates (e.g., see Cahalan's study) and, as discussed earlier, Cahalan found that low turnout rates were associated with decreased accuracy in responses.

Results for all four methods appear to be mostly similar on the registration question, with the random response method having the highest percentage of correct responses and the telephone method the lowest. For the primary election question the reverse was true, with the random response technique having the highest percentage of distortions and the telephone method the lowest.[8] However, no significant method effect overall was found in this study.

A telephone survey produced a higher percentage of accurate responses to a voting question (79%) than did face-to-face interviews (71%) in Rogers' (1976) study of residents in two New York City community planning districts (see Table 3.6). All interviews were conducted between March and July 1974 and concerned voting in a 1973 mayoral election.

The telephone sample contained a slightly higher percentage of actual voters than the face-to-face interview sample (45 versus 41%). Actual voters are usually unlikely to provide a false report. Four percent of those interviewed face-to-face did understate their voting as opposed to only 1% of the telephone sample. The telephone method also elicited a higher percentage of admissions of not having voted than the face-to-face interview method (64 versus 57%).

---

[8]See footnote 4 in this chapter.

Summary and Conclusions

1. For the 66 questions concerning comparatively nonthreatening topics, accuracy levels ranged from approximately 24 to 100%. This wide variation suggests that many factors other than question topic influence response validity.

2. Factors indentified by the primary authors, or explored in this investigation, with respect to their possible effect on the accuracy of individual's responses include:

    a. Whether the respondent ever had the requested information.
    b. The length of the recall period, or the recency of the event.
    c. The salience of the behavior.
    d. Related experiences of the respondent which may create interference effects or distortions in recall.
    e. Memory reconstruction, based on a need for consistency between behavior and attitudes, beliefs, or self-image.
    f. Social desirability or self-presentation concerns, conformity to ideal norms.
    g. Method. Considerations include that questionnaires may be comparatively impersonal. In-person interviewers may be able to probe and motivate.
    h. Question clarity.
    i. Particular characteristics of the respondents included in the survey, for example, demographic characteristics or the behavior patterns of the respondents.
    j. Acquiescence response set.
    k. Motivational variables, such as interest in the subject matter or in participating in the survey.
    l. The ability to check records or consult with other people.
    m. Question sensitivity.
    n. Anonymity of the respondents.
    o. The amount of specificity required in the response, for example, the exact number versus estimates or approximations, guided, perhaps, by categories provided.
    p. Whether proxy respondents were used.
    q. Forewarning that responses would be validated.

3. The effect of particular factors on response accuracy may be interactive. More accurate responses to particularly sensitive questions, for example, may be obtained with the comparatively impersonal questionnaire, but only if the respondent remains anonymous.

4. The prevalence of a behavior within the group of respondents can affect the overall level of truthfulness obtained. If the incidence of performance is high and the behavior is socially desirable, for example, truthful "yes" responses are highly probable.

5. Individuals' tendency to be truthful, as opposed to being a relatively enduring personal characteristic, may depend on the situation, or even on the particular question posed. (This issue is explored in Chapter 7.) This possibility underscores the importance of identifying the particular survey or question characteristics which affect respondents' ability or willingness to be truthful.

4

Reports on Sensitive Topics

Reports of Alcohol-Related Behaviors[1]

Locander *et al.* (1976), again with an aim of comparing the face-to-face interview, telephone, questionnaire, and random response survey methods, identified a sample of persons who had been charged with drunken driving within about a 1-year period prior to the survey and asked them if they had been so charged (see Table 4.1). The percentages of accurate responses were low for all techniques, from 46 to 65%.[2] Like the questions on absenteeism, this question concerned a socially undesirable behavior and generated large numbers of underreports.

Sobell, Sobell, & Samuels (1974) asked each of 70 men who had voluntarily admitted themselves to an alcoholism treatment program to report the total number of times they had been arrested for public drunkenness and for driving while intoxicated (DWI), whether they had ever been imprisoned in a state or federal penitentiary, and whether they were currently on formal probation. Respondents were queried on two separate occasions for the same information, once by the questionnaire method and the second time by means of a face-to-face interview, thereby giving the respondents an opportunity to change their responses.

Only 39% accurately reported their public drunkenness arrests (see Table 4.1). Contrary to expectations, respondents tended to overreport the number of arrests in this category. For DWI arrests, 63% of the responses were accurate, and distortions were mainly underreports. Of the 11 respondents who

---

[1]Questions directed to individuals who were described as alcoholics, or who can reasonably be assumed to have drinking problems, are presented separately rather than included with deviant behavior items because of the possibility that alcoholics constitute a distinct group in terms of their willingness or ability to be truthful.

[2]See footnote 4 in Chapter 3.

Table 4.1 Accuracy of Reports of Alcohol-Related Behavior

Study	Sample description	Method	Response rate (%)	Information requested	Number asked	Criterion	Accurate responses (%)	Over/under (%)
Locander et al. (1976)	249 Individuals identified through public records as having been "charged with drunken driving not less than 6 months or more than 12 months from the starting date of the study" (p. 270).	Face to face	57.1 (N = 36)	Whether charged with drunken driving in the last 12 months	30[a]	Public records	53	–/47
		Telephone	77.8 (N = 49)	Whether charged with drunken driving in the last 12 months	46	Public records	54	–/46
		Questionnaire	47.5 (N = 29)	Whether charged with drunken driving in the last 12 months	28	Public records	46	–/54
		Random response	58.1 (N = 36)	Whether charged with drunken driving in the last 12 months	33	Public records	65[b]	–/35
Sobell et al. (1974)	70 Male voluntary admissions to an alcoholism treatment program, who had also volunteered to serve in a research study	Questionnaire and face to face on the same information	100 (N = 70)	Number of arrests for public drunkenness	62[c]	Official arrest records	39	35/26
				Number of DWI arrests	62	Official arrest records	63	15/23
				Ever been imprisoned in state or federal penitentiary	11[d]	Official arrest records	63.6	–/36.4
				Whether currently on formal probation	13[e]	Official arrest records	53.8	–/46.2
Sobell & Sobell (1978)	Voluntary outpatient alcoholics'	Questionnaire (group condition)	100 (N = 14)	Number of hospitalizations at Orange County Medical Center	14	Official records	78.6[g]	7.1/14.3
				Number of hospitalizations at Metropolitan State Hospital	14	Official records	92.9	0/7.1

Number of hospitalizations at all other California State Hospitals prior to July 1969	14	Official records	78.6	21.4/0
Number of arrests for public drunkenness	14	Official records	92.9	7.1/0
Number of arrests for being drunk in auto	14	Official records	100	0/0
Number of arrests for open container	14	Official records	100	0/0
Number of drunk driving convictions	14	Official records	42.9	50/7.1
Number of arrests for assault and battery	14	Official records	100	0/0
Number of arrests for other crimes	14	Official records	92.9	7.1/0
Number of convictions for reckless driving	14	Official records	57.1	42.9/0
Number of speeding tickets in California last 2 years	14	Official records	64.3	35.7/0
Number of times California driver's license was revoked	14	Official records	92.9	7.1/0
Number of times California driver's license was suspended	14	Official records	85.7	14.3/0
Number of arrests related to drugs	14	Official records	100	0/0
Number of burglary arrests	14	Official records	92.9	0/7.1

(continues)

Table 4.1 (*continued*)

Study	Sample description	Method	Response rate (%)	Information requested	Number asked	Criterion	Accurate responses (%)	Over/under (%)
				Number of petty theft arrests	14	Official records	92.9	0/7.1
				Number of robbery arrests	14	Official records	92.9	0/7.1
				Number of arrests for assault with a deadly weapon	14	Official records	100	0/0
				Number of arrests for disturbing the peace	14	Official records	78.6	14.3/7.1
				Number of times on probation	14	Official records	57.1	7.1/35.7
				Number of times on parole	14	Official records	100	0/0
				Whether currently on probation	14	Official records	92.9	0/7.1
				Whether currently on parole	14	Official records	100	0/0
				Whether currently possess a valid California driver's license	14	Official records	100	0/0
	Outpatient alcoholics, court referred for treatment	Questionnaire (group condition)	100 (N = 12)	Number of hospitalizations at Orange County Medical Center	12	Official records	91.7	8.3/0
				Number of hospitalizations at Metropolitan State Hospital	12	Official records	100	0/0

Number of hospitalizations at all other California State Hospitals prior to July, 1969	12	Official records	100	0/0
Number of arrests for public drunkenness	12	Official records	100	0/0
Number of arrests for being drunk in auto	12	Official records	100	0/0
Number of arrests for open container	12	Official records	100	0/0
Number of drunk driving convictions	12	Official records	41.7	50/8.3
Number of arrests for assault and battery	12	Official records	100	0/0
Number of arrests for other crimes	11[b]	Official records	63.6	0/36.4
Number of convictions for reckless driving	12	Official records	58.3	33.3/8.3
Number of speeding tickets in California last 2 years	12	Official records	75	16.7/8.3
Number of times California driver's license was revoked	12	Official records	91.7	0/8.3
Number of times California driver's license was suspended	12	Official records	50	50/0
Number of arrests related to drugs	12	Official records	91.7	8.3/0
Number of burglary arrests	12	Official records	75	8.3/16.7
Number of petty theft arrests	12	Official records	100	0/0

(continues)

Table 4.1 (*continued*)

Study	Sample description	Method	Response rate (%)	Information requested	Number asked	Criterion	Accurate responses (%)	Over/under (%)
				Number of robbery arrests	12	Official records	100	0/0
				Number of arrests for assault with a deadly weapon	12	Official records	91.7	0/8.3
				Number of arrests for disturbing the peace	12	Official records	91.7	8.3/0
				Number of times on probation	11	Official records	54.6	18.2/27.3
				Number of times on parole	11	Official records	90.9	9.1/0
				Whether currently on probation	12	Official records	75	25/0
				Whether currently on parole	11	Official records	100	0/0
				Whether currently possess a valid California driver's license	12	Official records	91.7	8.3/0
	Voluntary inpatient alcoholics	Questionnaire (group condition)	100 (N = 13)	Number of hospitalizations at San Diego County, California, Detoxification Center	13	Official records	69.2	0/30.8
				Number of hospitalizations at Metropolitan State Hospital	13	Official records	100	0/0
				Number of hospitalizations at all other California State Hospitals prior to July, 1969	13	Official records	61.5	23.1/15.4

Number of arrests for public drunkenness	13	Official records	100	0/0
Number of arrests for being drunk in auto	13	Official records	61.5	38.5/0
Number of arrests for open container	13	Official records	76.9	23.1/0
Number of drunk driving convictions	13	Official records	53.9	30.8/15.3
Number of arrests for assault and battery	13	Official records	69.2	15.4/15.4
Number of arrests for other crimes	13	Official records	23.1	15.4/61.5
Number of convictions for reckless driving	13	Official records	61.7	38.5/0
Number of speeding tickets in California last 2 years	13	Official records	92.3	7.7/0
Number of times California driver's license was revoked	13	Official records	84.6	7.7/7.7
Number of times California driver's license was suspended	13	Official records	53.9	30.8/15.4
Number of arrests related to drugs	13	Official records	100	0/0
Number of burglary arrests	13	Official records	92.3	7.7/0
Number of petty theft arrests	13	Official records	84.6	7.7/7.7
Number of robbery arrests	13	Official records	84.6	7.7/7.7

(continues)

Table 4.1 (*continued*)

Study	Sample description	Method	Response rate (%)	Information requested	Number asked	Criterion	Accurate responses (%)	Over/under (%)
				Number of arrests for assault with a deadly weapon	13	Official records	84.6	7.7/7.7
				Number of arrests for disturbing the peace	13	Official records	53.9	46.2/0
				Number of times on probation	13	Official records	38.5	23.1/38.5
				Number of times on parole	13	Official records	100	0/0
				Whether currently on probation	13	Official records	84.6	15.4/0
				Whether currently on parole	13	Official records	100	0/0
				Whether currently possess a valid California driver's license	13	Official records	92.3	7.7/0

[a]See footnote *n* in Table 3.1.

[b]See footnote *o* in Table 3.1.

[c]For this and the following question, represents the *N* of respondents for whom data were reported.

[d]Represents the number of respondents who had been imprisoned.

[e]Represents the number of respondents who were on formal probation.

[f]For all three groups, the following criteria were used for subject selection: "a) no evidence of alcohol withdrawal symptoms or alcohol intoxication at the time of the interview; b) no evidence of organic brain syndromes or a primary diagnosis other than alcoholism; and c) voluntary participation in the study" (Sobell & Sobell, 1978, p. 902).

[g]For all questions, for all three groups, "To be scored as valid, interview answers had to be identical with the record data" (Sobell & Sobell, 1978, p. 902).

[h]In all cases where *N* = 11, one respondent did not answer the question. The authors reported six instances of unanswered questions. However, in their tabular presentation of data, only five such instances were reflected, one of which is omitted herein since it was highly unlikely that the criterion used was valid.

had been imprisoned, 63.3% reported that fact. Thirteen men were currently on probation, but only 53.8% of them admitted this.

In general, it is possible that alcoholics would not report very accurately on alcohol-related arrests, either due to the state of intoxication at the time of arrest, which would possibly affect recall, or to the embarrassing nature of the incident. Underreports, then, are understandable. That not all public drunkenness arrests are reported on official records may explain the high number of overestimates for this category. The authors suggested that DWI arrests may have been reported more accurately because DWI arrests are more salient to respondents. DWI arrests are processed more slowly than public drunkenness arrests and are typically followed by communications from the State Department of Motor Vehicles.

A further consideration may be that respondents in this study were told that their reports would be used in making treatment decisions. Perhaps some respondents exaggerated arrests to emphasize their alcoholic background, thereby influencing treatment plans.

Another factor that may have affected the validity of the responses was the time span referred to in the questions, or the amount of recall involved. The respondents ranged in age from 25 to 64 years. The older subjects were required, then, to provide information about behavior over a large number of years. Information about the relationship between age and response accuracy, however, is not provided.

Sobell & Sobell (1978) compared the questionnaire responses of three types of alcoholics: voluntary outpatient, court-referred outpatient, and voluntary inpatient. Participants were asked a number of questions concerning previous hospitalizations, arrests, convictions, parole and probation experiences, speeding tickets, driver's license revocations and suspensions, and driver's license possession. Some questions concerned incidents over the respondent's lifetime, one concerned the past 2 years, and three referred to the present. Since each respondent group consisted of a very small number of persons (14, 12, 13), the findings must be interpreted with caution.

For the voluntary outpatient alcoholics, the percentages of accurate responses ranged from about 43 to 100%, with the highest number of inaccurate answers given to the question concerning the number of drunk driving convictions (see Table 4.1). The percentages of accurate responses for the court-referred outpatient alcoholics ranged from approximately 42 to 100%, with responses to the question on drunk driving convictions again having the lowest percentage of accuracy. The range of percentage accurate responses for the voluntary inpatient alcoholics was from 23 to 100%. The lowest number of correct responses for this group was to the question concerning the number of arrests for what was referred to as "other crimes."

Unlike most of the responses considered up to this point, inaccurate responses for these groups were commonly in what may reasonably be considered the socially undesirable direction. Although the high percentages of overstatements in many cases must be considered in terms of the small N's involved, the fact that the number of overstatements frequently exceeds the number of understatements needs explanation.

One possibility is that the criteria applied were inexact. Three different types of records were used: driver records from the California Department of Motor Vehicles (CDMV), official arrest records of the California Bureau of Criminal Identification and Investigation (CII) and the Federal Bureau of Investigation (FBI), and hospital records (for the first two questions). Concerning the CII and FBI records, the authors admitted, "The information provided by these records constituted a *known minimum* number of arrests for any given individual" (Sobell & Sobell, 1978, p. 902, emphasis added).

Another possible explanation for the departure from the pattern of providing socially desirable responses, or a factor that may be operating along with the use of invalid criteria, is that alcoholics differ from other groups in their response tendencies, or in their perceptions of social desirability.

In making comparisons, question by question, across the three groups, it does not appear that any one group is more accurate than the others. However, the mean percentage of accurate responses for these 24 questions was somewhat different for the three groups: 86.9% for the voluntary outpatients, 84.8% for the court-referred outpatient alcoholics, and 76.0% for the voluntary inpatients. Subjects in the voluntary inpatient group had a higher mean age than subjects in the voluntary outpatient and court-referred outpatient groups (44.5 years versus 38.4 years versus 34.2 years). They also had longer drinking problem histories (mean years = 16.8 versus 8.6 versus 3.6), more alcohol-related arrests (mean arrests = 19.5 versus 4.5 versus 4.5), and more nonalcohol arrests (mean arrests = 4.0 versus 1.2 versus 1.3). Problems of recall, then, may have been greater for the voluntary inpatients than for the others. Differences among the groups in levels of accuracy, however, also seemed to depend on the particular question asked, with each group having certain questions on which response accuracy was greater than for the other groups.

Reports of Deviant Behavior

In Ball's (1967) follow-up study of 59 formerly nonvoluntarily hospitalized Puerto Rican drug addicts, approximately 81% of the respondents either reported the first arrest indicated on the FBI records or an earlier arrest (see Table 4.2). The reports of earlier arrests were assumed to be correct since they concerned mostly minor or juvenile offenses, the latter of which were said to be typically not reported to the FBI. Only one of the respondents denied having been arrested. About 33% of the respondents accurately reported the total number of arrests, with most distortions being overstatements.

First arrests may be more salient and easier to recall than total arrests over a period of years. It would be difficult to draw any conclusions about the overreporters. Since some offenses do not get reported to the FBI, the overreporters could have been telling the truth. Concerning the underreporters, the authors stated that offenses omitted from respondents' reports were mostly minor.

Through a urinalysis, Ball checked the responses of 25 subjects to a question concerning current drug use. Admissions might have been perceived by respondents as potentially incriminating. Whether subjects were aware that they would be asked to provide a urine specimen is unclear. Ninety-two percent of the respondents told the truth, including five subjects who admitted drug use. Two persons' denials were contradicted by the laboratory test.

Ball pointed to possible problems in language, definition, and interpretation as sources of bias. However, he also believed that certain procedures followed in the study contributed to accuracy. These included the interviewer's understanding of the addict subculture and the absence of any association with a police authority.

In Hardt & Peterson-Hardt's 1977 study, 89% of the seventh through ninth grade boys surveyed were truthful about whether they had ever been ticketed or arrested by police (see Table 4.2). Approximately 22% of the respondents claimed that they had been arrested or ticketed at some time in their lives.[3] The percentage of overstatements slightly exceeded the percentage of understatements.

A possible explanation offered for the high rate of overstatements was that some boys were already 16 years old, and tickets received after the sixteenth birthday were not recorded in the registry that was used to validate responses. Also, some ticketing might have occurred in other counties. To test these possibilities, the authors compared overreporting by boys under 16 years of age who had lived in the county at least 3 years with all other boys. The incidence of overreporting was more than twice as high for the latter group.

———————————————

[3]Respondents were given four response choices: "in the last 7 days," "in the last 12 months," "over a year ago," and "never." For the purposes of this analysis, responses were assigned to one of two categories, either "ever" or "never."

Table 4.2 Accuracy of Reports of Deviant Behavior

Study	Sample description	Method	Response rate (%)	Information requested	Number asked	Criterion	Accurate responses (%)	Over/under (%)
Ball (1967)	59 Puerto Rican drug addicts who were formerly incarcerated at the U.S. Public Health Service Hospital at Lexington, Kentucky	Face to face	NA (N = 59)	Type, place, and age of first arrest	57[a]	FBI arrest records	80.7	0/19.3[b]
				Total number of arrests	58	FBI arrest records	32.8	37.9/29.3
				Drug use at time of interview	25[c]	Urine specimen analysis	92.0	0/8
Hardt & Peterson-Hardt (1977)	Seventh- through ninth-grade male pupils attending schools located in nine selected census tracts in a middle Atlantic city with a population of slightly under 250,000	Questionnaire	NA (N = 914)	Ever been ticketed or arrested by police	862[d]	Official county records of police contact	89	6.5/4.5
Clark & Tifft (1966)	45 Male undergraduate students in the discussion sections of an introductory sociology course at a major Midwestern university	Questionnaire (group condition)	89 (N = 40)	(Since entering high school, how often have you) Run away from home?	40	Interview with polygraph exam	100	0/0
				Attacked someone with the idea of taking his (her) life?	40	Interview with polygraph exam	100	0/0
				Attempted to take your own life?	40	Interview with polygraph exam	100	0/0
				Used force to get money or valuables from another person?	40	Interview with polygraph exam	95	2.5/2.5

Bribed or attempted to bribe a police officer or another type of official?	40	Interview with polygraph exam	95	5/0
Carried a razor, switchblade, or gun as weapon?	40	Interview with polygraph exam	92.5	7.5/0
Taken part in gang fights?	40	Interview with polygraph exam	92.5	5/2.5
Used or sold narcotic drugs?	40	Interview with polygraph exam	92.5*	0/5
Taken things of large value (worth more than $50) that did not belong to you?	40	Interview with polygraph exam	92.5	5/2.5
Broken into and entered a home, store, or building?	40	Interview with polygraph exam	92.5	2.5/5
Struck your girlfriend or wife?	40	Interview with polygraph exam	92.5	2.5/5
"Beaten up" on someone who hadn't done anything to you?	40	Interview with polygraph exam	90	5/5
Defied your parents' authority to their face?	40	Interview with polygraph exam	85	7.5/7.5
Taken a car for a ride without the owner's knowledge?	40	Interview with polygraph exam	85	2.5/7.5
Forced or attempted to force a female to have sexual intercourse?	40	Interview with polygraph exam	85	2.5/7.5

(continues)

Table 4.2 (*continued*)

Study	Sample description	Method	Response rate (%)	Information requested	Number asked	Criterion	Accurate responses (%)	Over/under (%)
				Driven a motor vehicle in an unauthorized drag race?	40	Interview with polygraph exam	80	5/15
				Witnessed a crime and neither reported it nor made sure someone else had?	40	Interview with polygraph exam	80	7.5/7.5
				Started a fist fight?	40	Interview with polygraph exam	80	17.5/2.5
				Purposely damaged or destroyed public or private property that wasn't yours?	40	Interview with polygraph exam	77.5	10/12.5
				Driven a car without a driver's license or permit (do not include driver's training courses)?	40	Interview with polygraph exam	77.5	2.5/17.5
				Falsified information while filling out an application form or report?	40	Interview with polygraph exam	75	0/25
				Taken things from someone else's desk or locker at school without permission?	40	Interview with polygraph exam	72.5	2.5/25

Study	Sample	Method	N	Behavior		Validation method		
				Gambled for money or something else with persons other than your family members?	40	Interview with polygraph exam	67.5	7.5/25
				Bought or drunk beer, wine, or liquor illegally?	40	Interview with polygraph exam	65	2.5/32.5
				Taken things of medium value (worth between $2 and $50) that didn't belong to you?	40	Interview with polygraph exam	65	2.5/32.5
				Driven a motor vehicle at extreme speeds?	40	Interview with polygraph exam	52.5	2.5/40
				Skipped school without a legitimate excuse?	40	Interview with polygraph exam	40	2.5/55
				Taken little things (worth less than $2) that didn't belong to you?	40	Interview with polygraph exam	32.5	5/62.5
Voss (1963)	15.5% Simple random sample of seventh grade pupils in Honolulu intermediate schools	Questionnaire, group condition (20–25 respondents per group)	100 (N = 620)	Whether committed delinquent acts	52[f]	Police department records	98.1[g]	–/1.9

(continues)

Table 4.2 (*continued*)

Study	Sample description	Method	Response rate (%)	Information requested	Number asked	Criterion	Accurate responses (%)	Over/under (%)
Robins (1966)	524 White adults who had, as children, been seen at a psychiatric clinic during a 6-year period (Jan. 1, 1924–Dec. 30, 1929). These adults were not more than 18 years of age at the time of referral to the clinic, had IQs of 80 or over, and had a clinic history of behavior problems. Also, 100 control subjects, for whom there was no evidence of serious childhood behavior problems, were selected from public school records according to a quota sampling method. The controls were white, had IQs of at least 80, and were similar to the clinic	Face to face	81.7 (N = 491)[y]	Ever been arrested (nontraffic arrest)	164[b]	Police records	59	–/41
				How many arrests altogether	97[i]	Police records	51.5[k]	0/48.5
				Ever served time	83[l]	Court and prison records	71	–/29
				How much time served altogether	59[m]	Court and prison records	71.2[n]	0/28.8

subjects with re-
spect to sex, age,
and socioeconomic
status. 23 Subjects
who had died be-
fore the age of
25 were then
eliminated.[o]

[a]There is no information provided as to why the N is not 59 in this and the following question.

[b]Refers to the percentage of respondents who reported arrests later than the first one indicated in FBI records (17.5%) and those who denied any arrests (1.8%).

[c]"Of the fifty-nine subjects, three refused to provide a urine specimen, five were readmissions to the Lexington hospital, twenty-two were interviewed in jail or while hospitalized in Puerto Rico, and twenty-nine were living at home. The most meaningful validity measure concerned this last group; an accurate comparison of the verbal report of addiction and urinalysis was feasible for twenty-five of these twenty-nine subjects" (Ball, 1967, p. 652).

[d]Excludes 27 questionnaires where the respondents could not be matched with official records, and 10 questionnaires of respondents who did not answer the question. What happened to the other 15 cases is not clear.

[e]The authors report that those individual percentages that do not add up to 100.0 are due to "inaccuracies arising from respondents misunderstanding the meaning of an item" (Clark & Tifft, 1966, p. 518).

[f]Represents the number of pupils who were known to the police prior to the study.

[g]Represents the percentage of respondents who reported committing at least one of the delinquent acts for which records indicated they had been apprehended by the police.

[h]Represents the number of personally interviewed subjects known to have been arrested (incarcerated).

[i]Includes 416 personal interviews and 75 interviews with relatives of either living or dead subjects. At another point, the author states that there were only 411 personal interviews. This latter number may reflect the exclusion of 5 interviews in which written questionnaires were used.

[j]Represents the number of respondents who admitted having been arrested (served time).

[k]Within a range. However, full information on the ranges used was not provided.

[l]See footnote b.

[m]See footnote j.

[n]See footnote k.

[o]At another point, the authors stated that 22 subjects were eliminated.

Overreporting may also be attributed to the questionnaire instructions, which stated in part, "Young people do lots of things that are good — but once in a while they break some rules. Some of our most famous people said they broke quite a few rules when they were growing up" (Hardt & Peterson-Hardt, 1977, p. 259). It may be that this last sentence not only reduced inhibitions concerning admissions, but also encouraged overreports.

Clark & Tifft (1966) questioned 40 male undergraduate students concerning how often (not at all, 1–2 times, 3–4 times, over 4 times) they had committed each of 28 deviant acts since entering high school. Initially the respondents as a group completed questionnaires in pencil. Each questionnaire had a number, which only the respondent could identify as belonging to him.

In the second phase of the research, respondents were asked individually to select their questionnaires, privately modify them in pencil as necessary to achieve 100% accuracy, and then take a polygraph examination on the final responses.[4] During the examination, if there was an indication of deception, the respondent was asked if he wished to make a change in his response. Any changes at this time were made by the examiner in ink.

Finally, respondents were examined on their final responses and all "successfully passed" (Clark & Tifft, 1967, p. 116), apparently meaning that there was no "noticeable polygraph response" (Clark & Tifft, 1967, p. 116). Initial responses had been recorded by the researchers, so it was possible to compare the first responses with prepolygraph modifications, and finally with the responses made during the polygraph. The criteria against which initial responses were compared were the final responses following the completion of the polygraph.

Clark and Tifft felt that the final responses represented a greater degree of accuracy than the initial responses. It is possible that the greater accuracy of the final responses resulted from the threat or actual administration of the polygraph examination which may have motivated more truthful replies. Also, respondents were given additional opportunities to reflect upon their choices, which may have aided recollection. Change in method, from group-administered questionnaire to personal interview, may also have increased accuracy.

The authors reported that all respondents modified their initial responses, either prior to the polygraph at the time of the interview (58%) or during the examination itself (42%). Seventy-five percent of the changes were in the direction of increasing the frequency of admitted deviance.

---

[4]The authors discussed the fact that under certain conditions polygraph data may be invalid. However, they did not believe that their findings were significantly affected by these conditions.

The percentages of accurate responses in the initial answers to the questionnaire ranged from 100% to about 33% (see Table 4.2). In general, greater accuracy was associated with more serious offenses. The authors stated that there was less opportunity to change responses on these items since the incidence of committing them, based on the percentages of respondents admitting the behavior, is low. Also, the serious offenses were probably more salient to the subjects and easier to recall. Where, based on final admissions, the percentages of respondents having performed a behavior were high, inaccuracy was greater (see Table 4.3).

The relationship between prevalence and the accuracy with which performance frequency was reported for these socially undesirable items, which we measured by means of a Pearson correlation, was significant and negative ($r = -.874$, $df = 26$, $p \leq .001$). The greater the number of respondents actually performing the behavior, the less accurately it was reported. As previously discussed, we found a positive relationship between performance and accuracy for the socially desirable behavior items included in Cahalan's (1968) report. The greater the number of respondents performing the behavior, the more accurately it was reported, since the possibility for overstatements was decreased.

Cahalan's and Clark and Tifft's findings are not strictly comparable because Clark and Tifft's data concerned reports of behavior frequencies, while Cahalan's questions required either a "yes" or a "no" response. Behavior frequencies may be more difficult to specify. The number of changes made in responses to Clark and Tifft's questions between the "not at all" category (denials) and the other categories was not reported.

For most of the 28 questions, inaccurate statements included both underreports and overreports. Most of the distortions, however, tended to be underreports, increasing in number as overall levels of accuracy declined. There were five exceptions, for example, a question on starting fist fights, where false reports were mostly overstatements.

Like Ball's (1967) subjects, Clark and Tifft's respondents were very truthful (92.5% accurate) on a question concerning the use or sale of narcotic drugs. However, the questions differed. Clark and Tifft asked about the frequency of past behavior; Ball's question concerned current use, where an admission would more likely be perceived as incriminating. Also, all of Ball's respondents had a history of drug use. At the time of the study, Ball concluded that 7 of the 25 respondents, or 28% of the group, were currently using heroin. In Clark and Tifft's sample, only 10% claimed to have used or sold narcotic drugs during the time period in question. So, truthful "no" responses would have been more likely (see Table 4.3) for Clark and Tifft. That their respondents were only about as accurate as Ball's is probably because accuracy in Clark and Tifft's study required the

Table 4.3   Comparison between Performance and Accurate Behavioral Reports for Clark & Tifft's (1966) Deviant Behavior Items

Information requested	Percentage claiming performance	Percentage correct reports[a]
Bought or drunk beer, wine, or liquor illegally?	95.0	65.0
Taken little things (worth less than $2) that didn't belong to you?	87.5	32.5
Driven a motor vehicle at extreme speeds?	85.0	52.5
Skipped school without a legitimate excuse?	85.0	40.0
Gambled for money or something else with persons other than your family members?	80.0	67.5
Driven a car without a driver's license or permit (do not include driver's training courses)?	62.5	77.5
Falsified information while filling out an application form or report?	57.5	75.0
Defied your parents' authority to their face?	57.5	85.0
Purposely damaged or destroyed public or private property that wasn't yours?	55.0	77.5
Taken things from someone else's desk or locker at school without permission?	47.5	72.5
Driven a motor vehicle in an unauthorized drag race?	45.0	80.0
Taken things of medium value (worth between $2 and $50) that didn't belong to you?	45.0	65.0
Started a fist fight?	22.5	80.0
Broken into and entered a home, store, or building?	20.0	92.5
Witnessed a crime and neither reported it nor made sure someone else had?	17.5	80.0
Taken a car for a ride without the owner's knowledge?	17.5	85.0
Struck your girlfriend or wife?	15.0	92.5
Forced or attempted to force a female to have sexual intercourse?	15.0	85.0
Carried a razor, switchblade, gun as a weapon?	12.5	92.5
Run away from home?	12.5	100.0
Taken part in gang fights?	10.0	92.5
Used or sold narcotic drugs?	10.0	92.5
"Beaten up" on someone who hadn't done anything to you?	10.0	90.0

(continues)

Table 4.3 (*continued*)

Information requested	Percentage claiming performance	Percentage correct reports[a]
Bribed or attempted to bribe a police officer or another type of official?	7.5	95.0
Taken things of large value (worth more than $50) that didn't belong to you?	5.0	92.5
Attempted to take your own life?	2.5	100.0
Used force to get money or valuables from another person?	2.5	95.0
Attacked someone with the idea of taking his (her) life?	0.0	100.0

[a]Percentage accuracy in initial answering of questionnaire. In their report, seven of these percentages, plus the percentages of over and understatements, do not add up to 100.0 due to "inaccuracies arising from respondents misunderstanding the meaning of an item" (Clark & Tifft, 1966, p. 518).

identification of correct frequencies rather than a simple admission or denial.

Of the 620 seventh grade pupils in Voss' (1963) study on the ethnic group distribution of delinquent behavior in Honolulu, 52 were previously known to the police, having been "apprehended" for various offenses. Ninety-eight percent of these pupils (all but one) reported at least one of the offenses recorded against them (see Table 4.2). This included 48 respondents who reported all offenses and 3 others who each failed to report one act but acknowledged all others. The one respondent who underreported only had one recorded offense. This individual denied ever having been taken to the police station.

The possible discrepancy between the questions asked and the criteria used to evaluate the accuracy of responses poses a problem in interpreting the Voss (1963) results. Pupils were asked whether they had committed specific delinquent acts. The responses were compared to police records of apprehensions, as opposed to adjudications or convictions. The pupils who failed to report recorded offenses may not have actually committed the offenses.

Robins (1966) studied the adult social and psychiatric adjustment of individuals who had been referred to a psychiatric clinic before the age of 19. He also surveyed a control group of adults who had not been referred and for whom there was no evidence of serious childhood behavior problems. Included in the face-to-face interviews were questions relating to arrests and incarcerations.

Of the 164 respondents known to have had nontraffic arrests, 59% reported that fact (see Table 4.2). Of this group, about 52% provided an accurate report of the number of arrests. With respect to incarcerations, 71% or 59 of the 83 subjects who had served time admitted that fact, and 71% of those 59 respondents correctly reported the amount of time served. For the questions on the number of arrests and the amount of time served, inaccurate reports were all understatements.

An explanation for some of the inaccuracy may be found in the interview situation, because certain interviews were conducted in the presence of relatives. The exact number of these interviews and the precise association of this interview situation with the accuracy of reports of arrests and incarcerations was not reported.

When subjects were grouped according to the number of arrests they had experienced, Robins found that the proportion of subjects who denied having been arrested decreased as the number of arrests experienced by the subjects increased. Similarly, the lowest proportion of subjects who denied incarceration occurred in the group of individuals who had served the most time. The author also added, "The easy admission of prolonged incarceration and multiple arrests by the chronically criminal may have occurred only because *half of them were in prison at follow-up*, which made total denial of a criminal record impossible" (Robins, 1966, p. 273).

Respondents arrested since age 30 were less likely to deny all arrests than subjects whose last arrest occurred before the age of 31 (33 versus 55%). Although Robins (1966) allowed that this may simply be attributable to forgetting, he also suggested that, perhaps "reform diminishes the willingness to report past antisocial behavior" (p. 273).

Consistent with this explanation, juvenile arrests were more frequently denied by those who had not been arrested since the age of 18 than by those who had (64 versus 36%), and arrests between the ages of 18 and 30 were denied more often by those who had not been arrested since age 30 than by those whose arrest histories continued (66 versus 44%).

Reports of Sexual Behavior

Clark & Tifft's (1966) investigation, described earlier, included seven sexual behavior items. For these questions, the percentages of accurate responses ranged from 95 to 50% (see Table 4.4). It seems likely that the low figure of 50%, which concerned obscene materials, is at least partially attributable to the fact that the authors were not able to classify 30% of the responses as accurate or inaccurate because the respondents providing those answers were said to have misunderstood the meaning of this item. When those responses are excluded from this analysis, the percentage of accurate responses becomes about 71%.

Table 4.4 Accuracy of Reports of Sexual Behavior

Study	Sample description	Method	Response rate (%)	Information requested	Number asked	Criterion	Accurate responses (%)	Over/under (%)
Clark & Tifft (1966)	45 Male undergraduate students in the discussion sections of an introductory sociology course at a major Midwestern university	Questionnaire (group condition)	89 (N = 40)	(Since entering high school, how often have you)				
				Gotten a female other than your wife pregnant?	40	Interview with polygraph examination	95	2.5/2.5
				Visited a house of prostitution?	40	Interview with polygraph examination	95	2.5/2.5
				Had a steady girlfriend?	40	Interview with polygraph examination	90	2.5/7.5
				Had sex relations with a person of the same sex?	40	Interview with polygraph examination	80	5/15
				Had sex relations with a person of the opposite sex (other than my wife)?	40	Interview with polygraph examination	67.5	15/17.5
				Masturbated?	40	Interview with polygraph examination	65	5/30

(continues)

Table 4.4 *(continued)*

Study	Sample description	Method	Response rate (%)	Information requested	Number asked	Criterion	Accurate responses (%)	Over/under (%)
				Had in your possession pictures, books, or other materials which were obviously obscene and prepared to arouse someone sexually?	40	Interview with polygraph examination	50[a]	7.5/12.5
Udry & Morris (1967)	15 Black women, employed in menial jobs, who received positive urine specimen analysis reports indicating the presence of sperm	Questionnaire	100 (N = 15)	Whether had coitus within the past 24 hours	15	Three or more intact sperm in urinary sediment	80	—/20

[a]The authors report that these percentages do not add up to 100.0 due to "inaccuracies arising from respondents misunderstanding the meaning of an item" (Clark & Tifft, 1966, p. 518).

Inaccurate responses tended to be understatements of actual frequencies, with the greatest number of understatements associated with the question on masturbation. If we exclude the questions concerning obscene materials and having a steady girlfriend, which is a questionable sexual behavior item, then a negative relationship can be clearly observed between the percentages of accurate reports and the percentages of those claiming to have performed the behavior ($r = -.891$, $df = 3$, $p < .05$) (see Table 4.5).[5] As with the deviant behavior items, we found that the greater the number of respondents claiming to have performed the sexual behavior, the greater the inaccuracy in reports. Due to the small number of cases, however, this finding must be interpreted with caution.

Udry & Morris (1967) recruited 58 black women for participation in a study of urinary excretion of hormones. For a period of 90 days, each participant submitted a first-morning urine specimen along with a report slip indicating whether she had had coitus during the past 24 hours. Specimens and slips were dropped off at an unsupervised location and were marked by numbers only. A sample of these specimens was then analyzed for the presence of sperm. The presence of three or more intact sperms was taken as an indication that the women had had coitus within the past 48 hours.

Table 4.5   Comparison between Performance and Accurate Behavioral Reports for Clark & Tifft's (1966) Sexual Behavior Items

Information requested	Percentage claiming performance	Percentage correct reports[a]
Masturbated?	95.0	65.0
Had a steady girlfriend?	90.0	90.0
Had sexual relations with a person of the opposite sex (other than your wife)?	55.0	67.5
Had in your possession pictures, books, or other materials which were obviously obscene and prepared to arouse someone sexually?	50.0	50.0
Had sexual relations with a person of the same sex?	22.5	80.0
Visited a house of prostitution?	17.5	95.0
Gotten a female other than your wife pregnant?	7.5	95.0

[a]Percentage accuracy in initial answering of questionnaire. In their report, one of these percentages, plus the percentages of over and understatements, does not add up to 100.0 due to "inaccuracies arising from respondents misunderstanding the meaning of an item" (Clark & Tifft, 1966, p. 518).

_____

[5]For all seven items, $r = -.415$, $df = 5$, $p > .10$.

Forty-two positive laboratory reports were obtained for 15 women. These laboratory reports were compared with the women's written reports for the previous 2 days. For 12 respondents, the laboratory reports and the written reports were considered concordant; in all instances, the women reported sexual intercourse within the past 48 hours (see Table 4.4). Three women failed to report sexual relations during the reference period for certain of the positive laboratory reports.

The authors stated that the degree of accuracy was probably enhanced by a number of factors: the procedure, which provided anonymity to the respondents; the short time period (24 hours) covered in the written reports; and the fact that the women were not being asked to report on illicit sex acts. However, they also noted that at least some of the respondents may have suspected that the accuracy of their reports could be checked against the urine samples. Indeed it was the expression of this belief on the part of one of the subjects that provided the idea for this particular study.

Summary and Conclusions

1. For the 125 questions discussed in this chapter, accuracy levels ranged from approximately 23 to 100%. Even on sensitive topics, then, high rates of accuracy can be obtained.

2. Most of the factors listed in Chapter 3 (see Summary and Conclusions) as potentially affecting response accuracy were also identified in this review of questions on sensitive topics. Some additional factors discussed in this chapter include:

  a. The stated purpose of the survey.
  b. The setting in which the survey is conducted.
  c. The suspicion that responses could be checked.
  d. The level of threat posed by a question, including the fear of self-incrimination.
  e. The ability of the interviewer to establish rapport.
  f. Time to reflect.
  g. Whether a question calls for a "yes" or "no" response, as opposed to the specification of an amount or frequency.

3. Once again, we find that the factors appear to interact in their effect on accuracy.

4. In the case of socially disapproved behavior, overall accuracy for a group of respondents decreases with increases in the prevalence or frequency of performance of the behavior.

5

Reports on Financial Questions

Taxpaying Behavior

Hessing, Elffers, & Weigel (1988) examined the validity of individuals' responses to questions on taxpaying behavior, with tax collection records as the criterion.[1]

Using a complex procedure designed to assure the anonymity of respondents' replies, the authors surveyed individuals from two separate samples in 1984. The first group consisted of 71 Dutch taxpayers, labeled "evaders" (Hessing *et al.*, 1988, p. 407), known to have had their returns corrected by the tax collector for failure to disclose income or for taking unjustified deductions in each of two calendar years (1981 and 1982). Evasion was defined as "intentional underpayment of taxes" (p. 406). The total amount of the corrections for each year was at least 500 guilders. Further, two tax officials independently judged the returns for both years as exhibiting "fraudulent intent" (p. 407). This judgment was based on either "third party documentation of unreported income" (p. 407), or the "failure to justify deductible expenses when previously confronted" (p. 407). Further, respondents were drawn from a pool of "persons who had already been charged with evading taxes during both of the years under consideration and whose cases had already been settled, unprotested, prior to the beginning of this study" (p. 407). According to Elffers, Vrooman, & Hessing (1985), tax collectors and taxpayers may differ in their definitions of tax evasion. Therefore, any corrections made in categories that were known to be controversial were not included.

---

[1]Reference will also be made to reports of this study by Elffers, Weigel, & Hessing (1987), and Elffers *et al.* (1985), which contained some additional information.

The second group was comprised of 84 Dutch taxpayers who were labeled "nonevaders" (Hessing *et al.*, 1988, p. 407) in that their tax returns for both 1981 and 1982 were determined, following the initial routine review procedures at the time the returns were filed and two subsequent independent line-by-line audits, to require no corrections.[2]

Respondents in both groups were asked if they had failed to report income or had overstated deductions in each of the years in question. They were informed that answers would be compared with the tax collector's records but that this would be accomplished through a coding procedure to protect respondents' anonymity.

Just 25.4% of the evaders for 1981 and 28.2% for 1982 reported that they had either understated income or overreported deductions. On the other hand, in the nonevader group, 23.8% for 1981 and 20.2% for 1982 responded that they had failed to report income or claimed unjustified deductions (see Table 5.1).[3]

The extremely high rate of denials in the evader group suggests that these questions were perceived as threatening, in spite of the survey conditions. The authors believed that assurances of anonymity, the fact that the tax liabilities had already been exposed and settled unprotested, and willingness to participate were favorable conditions for obtaining accurate self-reports.

In addition, these events were also likely highly salient in that these respondents had been charged for 2 years. Also, respondents had been forewarned that their responses would be checked.

That the subject of income taxes in general is considered private or sensitive may account for the fact that only 20.8% of the evader group responded to the survey. Nonevaders also had a low response rate of 24.6%. Another equally plausible explanation for the low response rates, however, or at least a contributing factor, is that this was a survey introduced to potential respondents by mail. Individuals were then required to take an extra step and return a card indicating their willingness to participate.

In addition to question threat, other possible interpretations of the findings for the evaders bear examination. For example, certain evaders simply may not have agreed with the judgment of the Tax Inspectorate. Some possibly were unable to produce receipts for what otherwise would have been a legitimate deduction. Negative attitudes toward what was perceived as an unfair tax system may have motivated these evaders to participate, to have an

---

[2]Other researchers studying taxpaying and tax administration argue that many aspects of income tax assessment are both complex and uncertain enough that tax compliance does not have a clearly objective validating criterion comparable to those for the other topics included in this book. See for example, Kinsey, 1988; Smith, 1988; Long and Swingen, 1991.

[3]Data obtained from R. Wiegel.

Table 5.1 Accuracy of Reports of Financial Matters

Study	Sample description	Method	Response rate (%)	Information requested	Number asked	Criterion	Accurate responses (%)	Over/under (%)
Hessing *et al.* (1988)	Sample I: 342 tax evaders in the Netherlands	Questionnaire	20.8 (N = 71)	Did you, when filing your 1981 tax return, under-report your income or report unwarranted deductions?	71	Records of the Tax Inspectorate	25.4[a]	−/74.6
				Did you, when filing your 1982 tax return, under-report your income or report unwarranted deductions?	71	Records of the Tax Inspectorate	28.2	−/71.8
	Sample II: 342 nonevaders in the Netherlands	Questionnaire	24.6 (N = 84)	Did you, when filing your 1981 tax return, under-report your income or report unwarranted deductions?	84	Records of the Tax Inspectorate	76.2	23.8/0
				Did you, when filing your 1982 tax return, under-report your income or report unwarranted deductions?	84	Records of the Tax Inspectorate	79.8	20.2/0
Cahalan (1968); Parry & Crossley (1950); Crossley & Fink (1951)	See Table 3.1	Face to face	68.3 (N = 920)	Whether contributed or pledged money to Community Chest in Fall, 1948 drive	828[b]	Official records	62.2	37.8/0[c]

(*continues*)

Table 5.1 (*continued*)

Study	Sample description	Method	Response rate (%)	Information requested	Number asked	Criterion	Accurate responses (%)	Over/under (%)
Locander et al. (1976)	228 Individuals who "had all declared bankruptcy in the recent past" (p. 270)	Face to face	70.3 (N = 38)	Ever involved in bankruptcy	38[d]	Public records	68	-/32
		Telephone	68.9 (N = 41)	Ever involved in bankruptcy	41	Public records	71	-/29
		Questionnaire	59.3 (N = 35)	Ever involved in bankruptcy	31	Public records	68	-/32
		Random response	67.2 (N = 37)	Ever involved in bankruptcy	26	Public records	100[e]	-/0
Weiss (1968)	See Table 3.2	Face to face	NA (N = 1002)	Whether received money from welfare	680[f]	Official records	98	0/2
Ferber et al. (1969a)	Probability sample of 1100 families who owned 1419 savings accounts selected from a nonprobability sample of savings institutions in one major urbanized portion of the United States	Face to face, questionnaire[b]	70.6 (N = 777)	Savings account ownership	777[j]	Institutional records	54.2[g]	-/45.8
				Size of savings account	399[i]	Institutional records	10.4[i]	35.7/53.9
Ferber et al. (1969b)	Probability sample of 622 stockholders, drawn from a nonprobability sample of corporations in one major urbanized portion of the U.S.[k]	Face to face questionnaire[l]	68.5 (N = 426)	Common stock ownership	426	Institutional records	70.2[m]	-/30
				Number of common stock shares owned	290[n]	Institutional records	79.4[o]	7.8/12.8
Maynes (1965)	3270 Owners of savings accounts in the Netherlands Post Office Savings Bank, selected by	Face to face	78 (N = 2551)	Savings account ownership	2485[p]	Bank records	95	-/5
				Savings account balance in Oct, 1958	1700[q]	Bank records	NA	NA/65[r]

Study / Sample description	Method	Variable	N	Source		
means of a probability sampling method. Savings account owners were required to have only one known account at the bank, taken out in their own right, with a balance of 10 guilders or more. All respondents resided in a limited geographic area of the Netherlands.		Savings account balance in Jan., 1958	1700	Bank records	31[s]	NA/NA
David (1962) 50 Families who resided in a Midwest county and had the following characteristics: (1) a family head between 18 and 64 years of age; (2) some children under 18 years of age; and (3) received general assistance for at least 12 months prior to the date of the interview	Face to face 92 (N = 46)	Whether received public assistance income in 1959	46	Welfare office records	93.5	−/6.5
		Amount of public assistance income in 1959[t]	43	Welfare office records	41.9[u]	14/44.2
Ito (1963) 1795 Respondents from a U.S. National sample selected by means of a multistage sampling plan. Respondents were those who had made a new car purchase in 1954–1955 and had it financed, and for whom information from the lender was available.	Face to face NA	Amount of monthly payments for car	1757[v]	Lender reports obtained in interviews	65.5[w]	22.1/12.5
		Total amount of the loan (principal plus finance and insurance charges)	1794	Lender reports obtained in interviews	48	16.1/35.8
		Principal amount of the loan	1785	Lender reports obtained in interviews	28.5	24.1/47.5

(continues)

Table 5.1 (*continued*)

Study	Sample description	Method	Response rate (%)	Information requested	Number asked	Criterion	Accurate responses (%)	Over/under (%)
Hyman (1944)	War bond redeemers	Face to face	NA (N = 243)	Whether redeemed war bonds	243	NA	82.7	–/17.3
Weaver & Swanson (1974)	See Table 3.1	Telephone	56.5 (N = 339)	Monthly salary	278[x]	Records of the City of San Antonio personnel office	0.4[y]	84.5/15.1
Hardin & Hershey (1960)	Salaried insurance company employees, excluding those who were away from the office most of the time, those who worked part time or who worked in building maintenance, and company officers	Questionnaire Survey I: November 1957	NA (N = 283)	Any change in amount of pay in the past 6 months	241[z]	Personnel records	68	9[aa]/23[bb]
		Survey II: May, 1958	NA (N = 295)	Current gross salary	269[cc]	Personnel records	73[dd]	6/21
				Any change in amount of pay in the past 6 months	260	Personnel records	75	6/19
Lansing *et al.* (1961)	Study I: Addresses of owners of 133 individual savings accounts, selected from the records of a savings institution, so as to give representation to four different counties, three strata of account sizes, and three levels of account activity	Face to face	71.4 (N = 95)	Existence of savings account	77[ee]	Bank records	76.6	–/23.4
				Current size of savings account	59[ff]	Bank records	57.6[gg]	18.6/23.7
	Study II: Persons who had purchased a new car in 1956 and incurred a debt with that purchase, and who lived in a three county small city–rural area of Michigan	Face to face	NA (N = 25)	Total debt incurred at time of car purchase[hh]	25	State Motor Vehicle Registration Office records or county records	96[ii]	0/4

Study	Method / Condition	N	Dependent measure	n	Source	%	Ratio
Study III: Chicago residents, drawn from lists of people who had taken car loans	Face to face: Condition A—Long questionnaire/interviewer knew details of loan;	NA (N = 26)	Car loan taken	23[jj]	County and state records	73.9[kk]	−/26.1
			Amount of loan	17[ll]	County and state records	70.6[mm]	NA/NA
	Condition B—Short questionnaire/interviewer knew details of loan	NA (N = 30)	Car loan taken	27	County and state records	63	−/37
			Amount of loan	17	County and state records	94.1	NA/NA
	Condition C—Long questionnaire/interviewer did not know details of loan	NA (N = 19)	Car loan taken	15	County and state records	40	−/60
			Amount of loan	6	County and state records	83.3	NA/NA
	Condition D—Short questionnaire/interviewer did not know details of loan	NA (N = 17)	Car loan taken	14	County and state records	64.3	−/35.7
			Amount of loan	9	County and state records	88.9	NA/NA
Study IV: 33 respondents in a survey of consumer finances who had incurred a debt on a purchase of a new car	Face to face	NA	Whether new car purchase debt was incurred	33	State records	75.8	−/24.2
			Amount of debt incurred	25[nn]	State records	60[oo]	4/36

(*continues*)

Table 5.1 (*continued*)

Study	Sample description	Method	Response rate (%)	Information requested	Number askec	Criterion	Accurate responses (%)	Over/under (%)
	Study V: A probability sample of addresses of owners of individual or joint savings accounts in East Coast financial institutions. Each account was owned by one or two adults living in the metropolitan area and had a balance of $1000 or more at the time of selection into the sample.	Fall interviews: Face to face: Method A — Structured	76.8 (N = 63)	Existence of account	63	Savings institution records	78	–/22
				Account balance	40[p]	Savings institution records	57.5[qq]	17.5/25.0
		Method B — Unstructured	53.5 (N = 46)	Existence of account	46	Savings institution records	72	–/28
				Account balance	21	Savings institution records	63.6	4.5/31.8
		Face to face: Across both methods	64.9 (N = 109)	Existence of account 6 months ago	102[r]	Savings institution records	74	–/27
				Balance 6 months ago	55[s]	Savings institution records	63[u]	16.7/20.4
				Existence of account 1 year ago	86[uu]	Savings institution records	74	–/26
				Balance 1 year ago	45[w]	Savings institution records	71.2[uuw]	11.5/17.3
		Spring reinterviews: Face to face	73.4 (N = 80)	Existence of account in Fall, 1958	80	Savings institution records	86.3	–/13.8
				Best estimate of account balance in Fall, 1958	55[xx]	Savings institution records	58.2[y]	7.3/34.5
				Existence of account in Spring, 1959	78[zz]	Savings institution records	84.6	–/15.4
				Account balance on March 1, 1959	5C[AA]	Savings institution records	60[BB]	10/30

Study VI: Random selection of names of persons in two large cities who had borrowed cash from cooperating small loan companies	Face to face: Condition A — Respondent identified by name	73 (N = 32)	Whether made the cash loan	30[CC]	Lender records	30	—/70
	Condition B — Respondent's name not used	79 (N = 37)	Whether made the cash loan	34	Lender records	38	—/62
	Condition C — Respondent's name not used; sealed envelope	68 (N = 32)	Whether made the cash loan	30	Lender records	50	—/50
	Face to face: Over all survey conditions	DNA[DD]	Amount of payment per payment period	35[EE]	Lender records	82.9[FF]	8.6/8.6
			Total number of payments originally agreed upon	33[GG]	Lender records	63.6[HH]	12.1/24.2
			Number of payments made	33[II]	Lender records	57.6[JJ]	33.3/9
			Number of payments left to make	32[KK]	Lender records	43.8[LL]	9.4/46.9
Study VII: A probability sample of savings accounts in a savings institution. Only those accounts were kept with balances between $500 and $15,000 and which were owned by individual adults residing in the metropolitan area or its vicinity.	Face to face: Condition A — Respondent not paid; head of family preferred interviewee	67 (N = 26)	Whether account existed	26	Savings institution records	76	—/24
			Account balance as of January 1, 1959	17[MM]	Savings institution records	57.6[NN]	21.2/21.2
	Condition B — Respondent not paid; wife of head preferred interviewee	66 (N = 25)	Whether account existed	25	Savings institution records	70	—/30
			Account balance as of January 1, 1959	13	Savings institution records	88.5	0/11.5

(continues)

Table 5.1 (*continued*)

Study	Sample description	Method	Response rate (%)	Information requested	Number asked	Criterion	Accurate responses (%)	Over/under (%)
		Condition C — Respondent paid; head of family preferred interviewee	57 (N = 21)	Whether account existed	21	Savings institution records	82	−/18
				Account balance as of January 1, 1959	12	Savings institution records	85.5	7.3/7.3
		Condition D — Respondent paid; wife of head preferred interviewee	46 (N = 17)	Whether account existed	17	Savings institution records	68	−/32
				Account balance as of January 1, 1959	11	Savings institution records	75	0/25

a Data concerning the accuracy of responses to these questions were not contained in the referenced article, but rather were obtained in a personal communication with R. Weigel.

b Excludes 18 "don't remember" or "no answer" responses (= 2%), and 74 responses which could not be checked (= 8%).

c All "not gave" responses were assumed to be correct and not checked against records.

d See footnote *n* in Table 3.1.

e See footnote *o* in Table 3.1.

f Information on the rest of the sample is not presented.

g The researchers report that the data were weighted to correct for differences in sampling rates for originally sampled accounts (see their Table 1).

h Persons with an account size of $4999 or less were designated for direct interview, while those with an account size of $5000 and over were given a self-administered questionnaire in addition to an interview. However, the data were not reported according to this differentiation.

i Represents the number of respondents who reported the existence and size of accounts for which validating information was available. The researchers report that the data were weighted to correct for differences in sampling rates among families and for differences in response rates. Also excludes one institution in which a search for other accounts held by owners of originally sampled accounts was conducted, but no search was conducted for accounts owned by other family members (see their Tables 2 and 3).

j To the exact dollar.

k Excludes 36 cases found to be ineligible (deceased, abroad, etc.). Actually, this number represents batches of stock, being the "total number of shares in a given institution owned by a particular person or combination of persons." Only a very small percentage of stockholders (3.4% of the original sample) owned more than one batch.

[i]"Persons with holdings of 99 shares or less (approximately 60% of the original sample) were interviewed directly; while those with holdings of 100 or more shares (approximately 40% of the original sample) were designated for a combination interview/self-administered questionnaire procedure. However, the data were not reported according to this differentiation.

[j]"The researchers indicate that these data were "weighted to correct for differences in sampling rates, but not for differences in response rates." (See their Table 1).

[k]"Represents the number of respondents who both reported stock ownership and provided information on the number of shares. The researchers indicate that these data were "weighted to correct for differences in sampling rates among families and for differences in response rates" (see their Table 6).

[l]"To the exact number.

[m]"Sixty-six respondents were dropped from the sample either because it was discovered that they owned more than one account at Post Office Savings Bank or where the wrong person was interviewed. Thirteen "wrong interviews" were not caught in time to be excluded from analysis.

[n]"For this and the following question, represents the number of respondents who both acknowledged ownership and provided information on their account balances.

[o]"Respondents were assigned to one of 17 categories according to the mean actual account balance, such that there were approximately 100 respondents in each group. The percentage underestimating their balance in each group was reported. The figure reported above was calculated by adding the number of respondents underestimating across categories and then dividing by the number of actual respondents. According to the author, "An 'underestimate' exists where the reported balance is exceeded by the actual balance by one guilder or more" (see his Table 2).

[p]"Represents overall mean percentage calculated after grouping respondents according to size of balances and whether records were consulted, and then computing the percentage of correct responses in each category. A report was said to be correct if it was within 1 guilder of the actual balance.

[q]"Defined as including any cash payments and vouchers for food, rent, and utility bills. At one point, the author also included vouchers for clothing, but at another point, clothing was not mentioned.

[r]"Within 10%.

[s]"N's represent the number of respondents for whom lender and buyer reports were available.

[t]"Within plus or minus 1% error, for all percentage accuracy responses reported.

[u]"Sixty-one refusals (=18%).

[v]"To the exact dollar.

[w]"For this question in both surveys, excludes those respondents who were not employed 6 months prior to the survey and those for whom salary data and perceived change responses were not available.

[x]"For this question in both surveys, indicates reported change when there actually was no change.

[y]"For this question in both surveys, indicates reported no change when there actually was a change.

[z]"Number of respondents differs from total N, most likely due to some nonresponse to this particular question.

[aa]"To the exact dollar.

[bb]"Represents the number of accounts which could be checked, including "some secondary accounts which could be checked because they were in the same institution as the accounts originally selected" (Lansing et al., 1961, p. 13). The number of respondents associated with these accounts is not explicitly given.

[cc]"Represents the number of accounts which were reported.

[dd]"Represents accuracy within specified ranges, the sizes of which increased as account sizes increased.

[ee]"Determined by multiplying the reported number of monthly installment payments by their reported amount.

[ff]""Within a narrow margin of error" (Lansing et al., 1961, p. 23).

(continues)

Table 5.1 (*continued*)

dd For this question for all conditions in this study, excludes those respondents whose questionnaires were incomplete or for whom it could not be determined whether the loan in question was being discussed.

hh For this question for all conditions in this study, means reported the existence of the loan under investigation, whether primary loans—"loans taken out in connection with the original purchase of the car," or secondary loans—loans "taken out after the original purchase in which the car was put up as security" (Lansing *et al.*, 1961, p. 26).

ll For this question for all conditions in this study, represents those who reported the existence of the loan.

mmm For this question for all conditions in this study, indicates that either the "amount times number of payments is within 5 percent of recorded amount times number of payments," or the "amount borrowed is within 5 percent" even though "amount times number of payments is wrong by over 5 percent." Inaccurate responses were all those where the "amount borrowed is wrong by 5 percent or more by either calculation" (Lansing *et al.*, 1961, p. 28).

nnn Represents those who reported the existence of the debt.

ooo Applying the same criterion used in Study III, that is, within 5% of the recorded amount.

pp For both methods, represents the number of respondents who both reported the existence of the account and provided balance information.

qq For both methods, within $1000.

$rrrr$ Excludes 6 respondents whose accounts were not open on the specified date in Spring, 1958, and 1 respondent who was not asked the question" (Lansing *et al.*, 1961, p. 87).

ss See footnote pp.

tt See footnote qq.

uuu Excludes 22 respondents whose accounts were not open on the specified date in Fall, 1957, and 1 respondent who was not asked the question" (Lansing *et al.*, 1961, p. 87).

vv See footnote pp.

$wwww$ See footnote qq.

xx Represents the number of respondents who both reported the existence of the account and provided balance information.

yy Within $1000.

zz Excludes 2 respondents whose accounts were closed out by March 1, 1959.

AA See footnote xx.

BB See footnote yy.

CC Some respondents were lost in all conditions in this study, as by the time they were interviewed the loan was no longer outstanding.

DD Does not apply.

EE Represents the number of respondents from the total number of 37 who reported the cash loan for which information from lending records was available.

FF Within less than $5.

GG See footnote EE.

HH Within 2 payments.

II See footnote EE.

JJ See footnote HH.

KK See footnote EE.

LL See footnote HH.

MM For all conditions, represents the number of respondents who both reported the existence of the account and provided balance information.

NN For all conditions, within $1000.

opportunity to express these attitudes. In this case, negative attitudes toward the system would be highly correlated with evader denials, but this possibility was not explored by the authors.[4]

Regarding failure to agree with the Tax Inspectorate's judgment, it would be important to know when charges were made against the respondents. Were charges for both years made at the same time? Were the charges for 1981 made prior to or after the 1982 return was completed? If the charges for both years were made after the 1982 return was completed, then respondents may only then have learned about the discrepancy between the tax collector's and their interpretation of tax laws.

Given the stringent criterion used by the authors in selecting evaders, however, including that controversial categories were excluded, it is unlikely that this explanation, that is, disagreement with the Tax Inspectorate, would account for more than a small number of the denials.

Another possibility is that many respondents in the evader group, in answering the survey questions, considered their intentions when filling out their tax returns. If the underreporting of income or the reporting of unwarranted deductions was not intended, then respondents may have denied the behavior. Even though the specific questions put to respondents concerning their taxpaying behavior did not use the term *evasion* — which is perhaps commonly thought of as a deliberate act — many questions earlier in the survey made that explicit reference. Subjects may have been sensitized to think in terms of evasion as opposed to unintentional noncompliance. However, the authors attempted to exclude instances of unintentional noncompliance through the multiple criteria used to select individuals into the sample. Therefore, a reasonable conclusion is that at most only a few of the denials can be explained in this way.

What appears to have been a potentially more serious threat to the validity of responses concerns the possibility that respondents in the evader category, through various perhaps complex psychological processes, may have come to believe that they either did not intend to or actually did not evade paying taxes. These distortions in recall may result, for example, from the incongruence between perceptions of self as a good citizen and person and, at the same time, perceptions of self as a lawbreaker. As Cahalan (1968) noted:

> If the question permits the respondent to misinterpret or reconstruct his memories so he can give a response that is more con-

---

[4]Respondents were asked to rate the "fairness of treatment received from tax authorities" (Elffers *et al.*, 1987, p. 323). However, judging from the report, the relationship between this measure and respondents' answers to the tax behavior questions was not assessed for the evader group only. Rather, Elffers *et al.* (1987) computed a correlation between the two measures for the total group of respondents, including evaders and nonevaders.

> gruent with his own self-respect than the actual facts would be, he
> may tend to rewrite history more in line with what he thinks he
> ought to have done than with what he actually did. [pp. 609–610]
>
> Further, it may well be that certain questions on past behavior
> simply do not lend themselves to accurate measurement through
> survey research approaches, not because people do not want to
> tell the truth to others, but because they sometimes cannot tell the
> truth to themselves. [p. 621]

Being charged with tax evasion and the failure to protest these charges may have initiated a process of rationalization and denial.

One possible problem with this interpretation is that the evaders had corrections made for two consecutive years. It would probably be more difficult to deny two events of the same type except, again, if the charges for both years were made at the same time or if charges for 1981 were made after the 1982 return was completed.

To speculate about the motivations of the rather sizeable number of nonevaders who admitted failing to report income or taking unjustified deductions is perhaps more difficult. Again, if the criterion used was valid, then these individuals were probably bragging. This suggests that question threat was an issue only for the evaders, while for the nonevaders an admission served a positive function, perhaps enhancing status or conveying an "image of financial ingenuity" (Hessing *et al.*, 1988, p. 411). Lying in the context of this survey may have allowed these respondents a public self-presentation consistent with their private views on the subject.

Of course, another possibility is that these nonevaders were telling the truth; that is, they actually were evaders but were clever enough to conceal this fact. Then, the evasion would clearly have been intentional.

It is difficult to believe that all those who were able to hide their evasion would now admit to it in a survey. In fact, it seems more likely that they would be motivated to continue hiding their acts. Of course, it is possible that this 20% represents all those now willing to admit, indeed perhaps boast about, not getting caught. Yet to get 20% admissions suggests that a much larger percentage of this carefully selected sample of nonevaders were actually evaders, a conclusion which seems incredible.

An additional analysis performed by the authors concerning other items included in the survey is important to consider because it has direct relevance for the interpretation of responses to the taxpaying behavior questions.

In the mail introduction to the survey, potential respondents were told that the study concerned attitudes toward the tax system. They had time to consider their exact attitudes and were obviously willing to express them. In addition to the questions on taxpaying behavior, individuals in the two groups responded to items designed to measure first, attitudes toward concealing income, declaring false deductions, and tax evasion in general; second, perceptions of the frequency of tax evasion among relatives or friends, the anticipated reactions of significant others toward the respondent's hypothetical tax evasion, and the consequences perceived to be associated with tax cheating generally; and third, three personality characteristics believed to be associated with deviant behavior.

The questions on attitudes and what the authors called "subjective norms" (Hessing *et al.*, 1988, p. 410) preceded the questions on behavior. This might have caused individuals to consider their attitude and perceived norm statements when responding to the behavior questions. Perhaps respondents felt that a disparity between attitudes and actions would not only result in an inconsistent self-presentation, a possibility considered by the authors, but would also make their survey responses less credible. For example, some nonevaders may have had positive attitudes toward evasion and perceived it as a common practice with a generally low probability of detection. However, on a personal level, the perceived level of risk may have been high enough to inhibit the actual behavior. Lying in the context of this survey by falsely claiming to have cheated would have allowed these persons a self-presentation consistent with their expressed views on the subject.

Conversely, it is possible that individuals considered their behavior, or their beliefs about their behavior, when answering the attitude and perceived norm statements. For example, those evaders who denied cheating, either not admitting it to themselves or unwilling to disclose it publicly, may have expressed attitudes and perceptions consistent with their denials and their beliefs about the private nature of the subject. However, as noted by the authors, the personality measures would not have been affected by this process because these measures did not explicitly refer to tax evasion.

The authors' analysis of the relationships between the attitude, subjective norm, and personality measures and the respondents' self-reported and actual evasion status is in line with this consistency hypothesis and also provides support for the conclusions reached in the discussion in our report (see Table 5.2). These conclusions are that the respondents were mainly correctly classified as evaders or nonevaders and that the obtained inaccuracy for the former group resulted from denial, either public or private, and for the latter from bragging or a need for consistency in self-presentation. Given the scoring system used in the study, and accepting the measures as at least face valid, these explanations would predict the exact pattern of relationships found by the authors.

Additional analyses performed by the authors further support the consistency in self-presentation hypothesis (Hessing, Elffers, & Weigel, 1987). The authors calculated mean scores on their attitude toward tax evasion and

Table 5.2 Correlations between Tax Evasion and Measures of Attitudes, Subjective Norms, and Personality Attributes

	Tax evasion measures		
Psychological variables	2-Year self-report[a]	Documented status	Amount of taxes evaded[b]
Attitudes			
A_{act}[c]: Underreporting income	.25**	.07	.04
(M = 10.5; SD = 5.6)			
A_{act}: Unjustified deductions	.19*	.12	.10
(M = 11.1; SD = 6.3)			
A_{act}: Tax evasion	.28**	−.03	.00
(M = 2.4; SD = 0.9)			
Attitude toward tax evasion index	.30**	.07	.01
Subjective norms			
Perceived frequency	.22**	.09	.00
(M = 1.6; SD = 0.8)			
Social support	.22**	.01	.07
(M = 2.2; SD = 0.8)			
Negative consequences	.33**	.03	−.02
(M = 8.9; SD = 3.4)			
Perceived normative support index	.33**	.06	−.04
Personality Attributes			
Alienation	−.10	.22**	.29**
(M = 25.2; SD = 7.1)			
Tolerance of illegal behavior	.01	.18*	.22**
(M = 32.7; SD = 5.1)			
Competitiveness	−.05	.17*	.20**
(M = 25.0; SD = 7.6)			
Self-serving orientation index	−.07	.28**	.36**

Source: Adapted from Hessing *et al.*, 1988, Table 2, p. 410; Copyright © 1988 by the American Psychological Association. Adapted by permission.

Notes: *p < .05; **p < .01

[a]The 2-year self-report represents the sum of respondents' self-report scores for 1981 and 1982. No appreciable differences emerged when the analysis was repeated using the separate 1981 and 1982 reports as behavioral criterion variables instead of the 2-year report. The variable was coded 0 = negative responses to both taxpaying behavior questions; 1 = positive response to one taxpaying behavior question; and 2 = positive responses to both taxpaying behavior questions.

[b]Amount of taxes evaded refers to the average amount of corrections assessed against the respondent's tax return for the two years under consideration.

[c]A_{act} = attitude toward the act measures. Sample N = 155. For ease of comparison, Pearson product–moment correlation coefficients are presented throughout, although some variables were dichotomously or trichotomously scored. Substitution of point–biserial correlations or Spearman's rho where appropriate yielded virtually identical results.

perceived normative support indices for four groups of survey participants: evaders who reported misrepresentation, nonevaders who reported misrepresentation, evaders who denied misrepresentation, and nonevaders who denied misrepresentation.[5] On both indices, mean scores for the groups who reported misrepresentations were similar. The mean scores for these groups were significantly different from the mean scores for the two denier groups. Scores for the groups who denied misrepresentation were also similar. Judging from the mean scores on these indices for these groups, self-reported evaders had more positive attitudes toward tax evasion and perceived more social support for evasion behavior than did those who denied evading taxes.

For the personality variable index, however, which was presumably not associated with taxpaying behavior, similar mean scores were obtained for both groups of evaders. These scores were significantly different from the mean scores obtained for both groups of nonevaders, which were highly similar to each other.

One concern with the relationships found in Table 5.2 is that the number of inaccurate nonevaders is small, and associations for this group may not have greatly affected the overall results. Since evaders and nonevaders apparently differed in their response motivations, an analysis for each group seems appropriate. Also, the correlations obtained, although significant, are low. Although these low correlations may be partially attributable to an imperfect categorization of respondents as evaders or nonevaders and also attributable to an imperfect measurement of the psychological variables, separate analyses may prove useful for further interpretations of the study's results.

These findings on Dutch taxpayers have relevance for estimates of the validity of data obtained in surveys of taxpayers in the United States. Assuming that the populations in the two countries are comparable, that the evaders sampled are similar to evaders in general, and that the Dutch and the U.S. tax systems are similar, consider the implications. According to Hessing *et al.* (1988) the Internal Revenue Service estimates that evasion occurred on more than 35% of the returns sampled.[6] This, then, excludes failure-to-file evasion. Not all of the occurrences would meet the stringent tests imposed by the authors, but one purpose of their criteria was to establish intention.

In a random sample of 1000 taxpayers, there would be 350 evaders and 650 nonevaders. Approximately 27% of the evaders or 95 persons would acknowledge evading taxes. But about 22% or 143 nonevaders would also claim evasion. The total percentage of respondents categorized as evaders would be 23.8%. This figure is similar to the median percentage of respondents (20%) who admitted evading taxes in the nine surveys on federal taxpaying behavior reviewed by Kinsey (1984). Conclusions drawn from any individual-

---

[5]It is assumed that the authors mean in either year.

[6]The source of this datum was not provided, nor was the year for which this estimate was made. According to the information provided by Kinsey (1984), this figure is consistent with IRS estimates of undercompliance, whether intentional or nonintentional, in recent years.

level analyses would be incorrect, since about 60% of the evaders would actually be nonevaders.

Individual-level analyses of taxpayer survey data might be even more problematic than suggested above, because evaders are probably concentrated in specific population groups and also because they may be harder to reach with ordinary survey techniques than nonevaders. Their true numbers would then be underrepresented in a random sample or even in a probability sample. The overrepresentation of nonevaders would result in an even greater proportion of false positives. For a full discussion of these methodological issues, see Skogan (1981).

Other Financial Questions

In Cahalan's (1968) study, the Denver respondents were asked whether they contributed or pledged money to the Community Chest in a fund-raising drive the previous fall. Only about 62% of the respondents were truthful; 38% falsely claimed to have contributed (see Table 5.1). Again, Cahalan argued that responses to questions concerning past behavior are more likely to be inaccurate since memory can be reconstructed to be more congruent with a respondent's self-image. Parry & Crossley (1950) suggested that social pressures were a factor.

Locander et al. (1976), using four methods, questioned individuals who had all recently declared bankruptcy about whether they had ever been involved in bankruptcy. The random response method produced 100% accurate responses, while the other three methods, face to face, telephone, and questionnaire, all produced about 70% accuracy (see Table 5.1).[7] The authors concluded that the random response method reduced underreporting of socially undesirable acts. However, they also stated that bankruptcy may not be perceived by all persons as socially undesirable. For some, it may represent a shrewd business tactic. No significant method effects were found over all questions included in this study.

Ninety-eight percent of Weiss' (1968) welfare mother respondents reported having received money from welfare (see Table 5.1). Weiss attributed this high rate of accuracy to two facts: One, that half of the interviews included an introductory statement which described this as a survey of welfare mothers; and, two, that the previous questions assumed that the respondent was a welfare recipient.

Ferber et al. (1969a,b) conducted two reverse record check studies specifically designed to ascertain the validity of self-report data concerning savings

---

[7]See footnote 4 in Chapter 3.

account ownership and common stock holdings. In both studies, the reference date used was about 6 to 9 months prior to the interview date.

Almost one-half of the respondents denied owning any savings account (see Table 5.1). Of the 421 respondents who reported their accounts, only 410 were also willing to report the account size. Of these, validating information was available for 399 respondents. Only about 10% of these reported their account size to the exact dollar, with over half of the distortions being understatements.

On the existence of accounts question, the authors suggested that memory was a factor contributing to inaccuracy since small accounts tended to go unreported. Problems with recall may have affected accuracy on reports of the size of accounts, because respondents were asked to provide information on their accounts for a reference date about 6 to 9 months in the past. Also, the standard for accuracy used—to the exact dollar—was demanding.

For common stock holdings, reports were more accurate. Seventy percent of the respondents acknowledged ownership (see Table 5.1). Of those who were also willing to provide information on size, meaning the number of common stock shares owned (only 11 respondents declined), almost 80% were truthful. The dramatically higher rate of accuracy in responses to the question on the number of stock shares owned as compared to the question on the size of savings accounts may possibly be attributable to the greater stability in the number of shares owned versus the dollar amount in a savings account.

In both of the Ferber et al. (1969a,b) studies, the interviewing unit was apparently the family rather than the originally sampled savings account or stock owner. Heads of households were apparently interviewed concerning all household members. Some inaccuracy, then, could have resulted from interviewing a nonowner, who may not have been aware of or familiar with the account or stock holding.

In Maynes' (1965) October, 1958 survey of savings account owners in the Netherlands, 95% acknowledged ownership (see Table 5.1). This finding sharply contrasts with Ferber et al.'s (1969a) finding, perhaps because in Maynes' study, account owners reported only for themselves and not for other household members. Also, respondents were questioned regarding current ownership as of October, 1958, whereas in Ferber et al.'s study, the reference date was many months earlier.

For current balance information, though, underreporting was high, even though respondents were encouraged to consult records. A tendency to underreport large balances and overreport small balances was found. Information on the percentage of accurate responses or overstatements was not presented.

Respondents were also asked to report account balances as of January, 1958. Only 31% of these responses were accurate. Data concerning the percentages of overreports and underreports were not provided.

Maynes suggested that interviewees wish to be perceived as "average men" (1965, p. 380) and will, therefore, respond to survey questions based on their notion of what represents "average." This explains the tendency to overreport small balances and underreport large balances, even when records have been consulted.

Interviewed some time in 1960 by David (1962), almost 94% of the families who had received general assistance acknowledged having received public assistance income in 1959 (see Table 5.1). Of this group, only about 42% accurately reported the amount, with 44% of the reports being understatements. This occurred despite the fact that, in this survey, assistance income was broken down into categories, and interviewers added the amounts reported. On the other hand, it may be difficult to remember amounts received in all categories, especially because most income was received in the form of vouchers.

In Ito's (1963) analysis of data from a 1956 study of consumer finances concerning loans made in 1954 or 1955 for new car purchases, almost 66% of the respondents correctly reported their monthly car payments (see Table 5.1). Most errors on this question were overstatements. Response accuracy was lower on a question about the total amount of the loan (48%) and lowest for reports of the principal amount of the loan (28.5%). Erroneous reports to the latter two questions were mainly underreports.

To account for the differences in reporting accuracy, Ito suggested that monthly payment amounts are more salient to respondents than either total or principal loan amounts. That total loan amounts were reported more accurately than principal loan amounts was explained by the fact that, at the time of the interview, interviewers did a consistency check between the amount and number of monthly payments and the total loan amount, presumably providing an opportunity for respondents to change their answers on the total loan amount.

Hyman (1944) interviewed, within 7 days following redemption, 243 persons who had redeemed war bonds. When the originally selected respondent was not home, the spouse was interviewed. How often this occurred is not reported. About 17% of the interviewees denied having redeemed the bonds (see Table 5.1).

In Weaver & Swanson's (1974) study discussed earlier, of 278 firemen and policemen asked about the amount of their monthly salary, only one reported it exactly (see Table 5.1). Confusion about deductions does not explain the inaccuracy because almost 85% of the distortions were overreports. The authors expected that respondents would be aware of their exact salaries since many had observed recent salary negotiations that had also been widely publicized. The authors conjectured that respondents may think more in terms of yearly salaries; but, when an additional 17 respondents were queried about their yearly salaries, none were correct and 15 were overstatements.

The most plausible explanation for these results is in the question itself. The authors recognized that they should have asked about salary "at this job" (Weaver & Swanson, 1974, p. 72), since reports were only checked against city records for policemen and firemen and respondents may have had additional part-time jobs.

Salaried insurance company employees were queried through a questionnaire by Hardin & Hershey (1960) in two surveys about pay changes. The survey focused on reactions to a technological innovation, and the questionnaires were administered just prior to, and again at some point after, the introduction of the innovation. A question on whether a respondent's salary had changed and how much it had changed in the past 6 months was included.

In the first questionnaire, 68% of the respondents provided correct reports, while 75% were accurate in the second questionnaire (see Table 5.1). Accurate responses were those in which no change was reported when there actually was no change, or when employees reported earning "much more now," "more now," "less now" or "much less now" and records confirmed a change, irrespective of the amount or direction. Therefore, some incorrect responses may have been counted as accurate. For example, some respondents may have reported earning "less now" while records indicated a salary increase; yet only change was measured, so the response would have been considered accurate. It appears, however, that only about two persons in the first survey and one in the second reported decreases in earnings. Most of the inaccurate answers were reports of no change when records indicated at least some change.

The first survey also included a question on current gross salary, to which 73% of employees provided correct responses, that is, to the exact dollar. Inaccurate responses were mainly understatements.

Lansing *et al.* (1961) conducted a series of seven studies designed to provide information concerning the amount of response error in surveys of financial data. Factors believed to have contributed to response error in each study were identified and discussed. Modifications to improve response accuracy were introduced into the succeeding studies.

In the first study, addresses of owners of individual savings accounts were obtained from the records of a savings institution. Apparently, the actual owners of the accounts were not specifically selected for interview. Rather, the interviewers were instructed to talk with the "proper respondent or spouse" (Lansing *et al.*, 1961, p. 14). Information on exactly who was interviewed is not given. Some error may have been introduced by interviewing persons other than account owners; nonowners may not have been familiar with the account (see the earlier discussion of the Ferber studies with the same problem and low accuracy).

Also, respondents were not asked to name the particular institution in which the account that they reported was located. Although account information was compared with bank records to check for a match, the authors admit the possibility of incorrect matches in some cases.

About 77% of the savings accounts were reported (see Table 5.1). Only about 58% of the reports of the account balances were accurate. Most distortions were underreports. Accuracy was determined by reference to specified ranges which increased as account size increased. For example, a report on an account with an actual balance of between $1 and $199 was accurate if it fell within this range. Larger accounts had wider ranges, so there was more leeway for response inaccuracy. For example, accounts between $10,000 and $24,999 had that wide range for judged report accuracy. Also, if the reports were outside the range, even by the smallest amount, the response was apparently considered inaccurate. In this case, a $25,000 response to a $24,000 account would be considered inaccurate, while a $15,000 response would be considered accurate.

The next three studies conducted by Lansing *et al.* (1961) concerned indebtedness for new car purchases. Subjects in the first of these studies were 25 persons from a three-county area in Michigan who had recently purchased a new car. In this study, the interviewer was fully aware of the purposes of the study and attempted to tape-record all of the interviews (whether or not surreptitiously is not reported).

Respondents were asked about the number and amount of monthly payments. Total indebtedness was calculated from the replies. Using this approach, for 24 of the respondents (96%), the total incurred debt for the car purchase was correct "within a narrow margin of error" (Lansing *et al.*, 1961, p. 23) (see Table 5.1). Discrepancies were attributed to different payment amounts in some cases for certain months, incorrect reports of the total number of payments, and rounding.

In the second study of car debt, interviewees were randomly assigned to one of four interview conditions, representing situations in which the interviewers either knew or did not know the amount of the loan, and where the questionnaire was either long or short. Addresses of Chicago residents who had purchased a car within about the past one and a half years were selected for interview. Whether the interview was taken with the recorded purchaser or some other person at the selected address is not clear. The loans in question were either the original car loan or a secondary loan, that is, a loan made after the car purchase where the car was used as security.

For each interview condition, data were presented on the accuracy of respondents' reports on whether the loan under investigation was taken and on the total amount borrowed. For the latter question, responses to a direct inquiry on the amount borrowed and also to questions on the total number and amount of payments were examined. The degree of accuracy varied somewhat by condition. Situations where the interviewer did not know the details of the loan and in which a long questionnaire was used produced the poorest results (see Table 5.1).

Further analysis revealed that a principal source of response error in this study involved the failure to report secondary loans. The authors determined that 36 of the loans in question were clearly primary loans, while 39 were secondary. About 89% of the primary loans were reported; about 81% of those had accurately reported balance information. These figures contrast with almost 44% of the secondary loans reported; 88% of those had balance information accurately reported. The authors reasoned that the questionnaire used may not have been appropriate to elicit information about secondary loans. Also, respondents may have been reluctant to discuss secondary loans because, in some cases, the loans resulted from difficulty making payments on the original loan. It should also be noted that all of the respondents, except one, who failed to report the loan in question, reported another loan.

The final study on car debts involved persons who had reported purchasing a new car, whose names were taken from the National Survey of Consumer Finances. Using state records, reports were checked and in 33 cases information was obtained on the existence and amount of debt. Of the 33 cases, 25 (almost 76%) reported the existence of the debt (see Table 5.1). Of this group of 25, 60% accurately reported the debt amount within 5% of the recorded amount, while 36% of the responses were understatements.

Lansing *et al.* (1961) compared these findings with the findings on primary loan reports from the Chicago residents' study of car debt discussed earlier. They concluded that the Chicago study results were superior because interviews focused on a limited topic; the Survey of Consumer Finances covered many topics.

In a fifth study, two different interview methods, structured and unstructured, were used to survey individuals regarding savings accounts. Addresses were obtained from financial institutions of savings account owners with balances of $1000 or more. These owners were reportedly asked for "by name" (Lansing *et al.*, 1961, p. 92), but the actual owners were not necessarily the respondents. Apparently, either the head of the household or the spouse was interviewed and asked to report for all family members.

An examination of the two instruments reveals that only respondents interviewed with the structured questionnaire were told that records could be consulted. Information was requested on account balances as of the first of the month in which the interview was conducted.

Seventy-eight percent of the respondents interviewed with a structured questionnaire versus 72% of those in the unstructured interview condition reported the savings account in question (see Table 5.1). The authors noted that some of the unreported accounts were owned entirely or in part by someone other than the respondent or spouse, presumably another family member or even someone outside of the family. These unreported accounts represented almost 14% of the total number of unreported accounts in the structured interview condition and about 39% in the unstructured interview condition.

An important difference in the two approaches is the percentage of those who reported the account who were also willing to report the account balance, 81.6% versus 66.7% for the structured and unstructured approaches respectively. Of those reporting the balance, 57.5% were accurate using the structured method, while 63.6% were accurate using the unstructured method. The authors suggested that the unstructured approach may have been threatening to the respondents and to the interviewers, since the interviewers were accustomed to a structured approach.

The respondents were also queried concerning family ownership of savings accounts 6 months prior and 1 year prior to the interview. For both questions, of those who had open accounts on those target dates, 74% acknowledged ownership (see Table 5.1). Almost 30% of the unreported accounts for the 6-months-ago date and 27% for the 1-year-ago date were owned at least in part by someone other than the respondent or spouse. Sixty-three percent of the interviewees who also gave balance information for the 6-months-ago date were correct in their reports, while the percentage correct for the 1-year-ago date was slightly over 71%.

The first interviews took place in the fall of 1958. In the spring of 1959, apparently using only one method, reinterviews were attempted. Respondents were again asked about savings accounts and balances as of Fall, 1958. Of the 80 persons who agreed to the second interview, over 86% reported the account. The 55 individuals who gave balance information were also requested to resolve any conflict between the fall and spring reports of the fall balance.[8] The revised report was called the "best estimate" Lansing et al., 1961, p. 69). Slightly over 58% of these respondents offered accurate "best estimates."

---

[8] However, 8 of the 55 did not report the balance during the fall interview. Apparently, their spring report was considered their "best estimate."

Of the 80 reinterviewees, 78 were associated with accounts that were still open in the spring of 1959. Almost 85% of those individuals reported the accounts, while 60% of those who reported spring balances were accurate.

A sixth study by Lansing *et al.* (1961) focused on the topic of consumer credit; persons who had borrowed cash from small loan companies were the subjects. The researchers considered this topic as private or sensitive. In order to obtain accurate reports, the researchers felt that the interview situation must be managed in such a way that it would be viewed as different, or governed by its own set of standards or norms. Respondents' perceptions of the guarantee of anonymity were considered a key factor for response accuracy. Procedures which provided greater assurances of confidentiality were presumably associated with greater response accuracy.

To test this hypothesis, sample addresses were randomly assigned to one of three groups. In Group A, respondents' names were known ahead of time, and interviewers were instructed to make sure that they had the right respondent by name. This manipulation, however, may not have been entirely successful, because interviewers were told that they could wait until after the interview to make this check.

Group B interviewers were told not to use the respondent's name in any way or at any time but to use nonobvious methods to ensure that the right respondent was being interviewed. In effect, Group A and Group B respondents may have been treated the same.

For Group C, in addition to not mentioning the respondent's name, some special techniques were used to increase motivation by heightening the perception of anonymity and creating a sense of the survey's usefulness to the respondent. For example, the financial data section in the interview, completed either by the respondent or by the interviewer, was designed to be detached from the rest of the survey, placed in a stamped envelope, sealed, and directly mailed to the Survey Research Center. Also, these respondents were given a special explanation about a report that would be sent to them, containing information obtained in the research about how the survey participants handle their financial affairs.

For acknowledging the existence of the cash loan in question, as of the first of the month in which the interview was conducted, the greatest accuracy was associated with Group C, where 50% of the respondents reported the specific loan, as opposed to 30% in Group A and 38% in Group B (see Table 5.1). Groups A and B were, then, similar in outcome. The authors concluded that the superiority of Group C can be attributed to the reinforcement of the assurance of confidentiality through the use of the sealed-envelope technique.

However, Lansing *et al.* (1961) also stated that in 9 of the 94 completed interviews the respondent was not the borrower and that replies were more accurate when the respondent was the borrower (11% of the former group reported the known loan versus 42% of the latter group). The distribution of these 9 cases across the three conditions is not reported. Consequently, the possible differential effect on accuracy cannot be determined.

A certain percentage of respondents in each condition who failed to report the loan in question reported other loans, either cash loans or installment purchases. The percentages who reported no loans were 13% for Group A, 18% for Group B, and 3% for Group C. The results of this comparison support the idea that Group C represented a superior interview condition.

Information was also presented on the accuracy of responses across all survey conditions to other questions about the cash loans. For example, of the respondents who reported the cash loans under investigation, correct replies were provided by almost 83% concerning the amount of payment per payment period, by close to 64% regarding the total number of payments originally agreed upon, by about 58% concerning the number of payments made, and by almost 44% to the question on the number of payments due (see Table 5.1).

The final study by Lansing *et al.* (1961) involved owners of savings accounts with balances between $500 and $15,000. Owners were assigned to one of four interview conditions which represented situations where interviewees were or were not paid for the interview, or where the head of the family, preferably the husband, or the spouse was interviewed.

The authors hypothesized that those who were paid would be more motivated to cooperate and, consequently, provide better information. Also, the authors wished to compare results where husbands versus wives were interviewed to ascertain whether there is a gain in accuracy corresponding to the extra effort expended to interview the husband. However, the authors also reported that a respondent other than the designated interviewee could have been interviewed if it was necessary. For example, if the husband was not available in the "head of the family" (Lansing *et al.*, 1961, p. 120) conditions, then the wife could have been selected. Also, if the wife was the designated respondent, the form could have been left with her overnight so she could consult with her husband. For these reasons, the authors refer to the designated interviewees as the "preferred" (p. 127) interviewees for that condition.

For all conditions, the sealed-envelope technique was used for financial data; the interviewer was instructed to take most of the responsibility for the form's completion. The interviewers were also instructed to avoid asking for the respondent by name.

One possible problem in interpreting the results of this study involves the amount of time between the interview and the reference date for account information. Respondents were questioned about account balances as of January 1, 1959. However, the authors noted that for those respondents who had new accounts, the target date was July 1, 1959.[9] That the July date was some-times used indicates that interviews were conducted 6 months or more after January 1, 1959. This situation introduces a possible recall factor.

Small differences in response accuracy were reportedly found among the four conditions, although apparently the best results overall occurred for the condition where the preferred respondent was the head of the family and was paid (see Table 5.1). In this case, 82% of the interviewees reported the account, and 85.5% of those who reported a balance provided an accurate report.

A comparison can also be made among the conditions as to whether balance information was provided by those persons reporting the account. The percentages of respondents who reported the account but refused to state the balance were 15% for Condition A (no pay, head of family preferred), 27.7% for Condition B (no pay, wife preferred), 35.3% for Condition C (pay, head of family preferred), and 8.3% for Condition D (pay, wife preferred). Most of the accounts that were *not* reported (57.7%) were accounts that were owned either entirely or in part by someone other than the respondent and spouse.

Lansing *et al.* (1961) suggested three broad categories of possible reasons for response error in reports of financial data: (1) motivational factors, affecting the willingness of respondents to provide accurate information; (2) problems in communication, where it may not be clear to the interviewee what is being asked or to the interviewer what is being reported; and (3) inaccessibility of the requested information, through inability to recall, distortions in memory, or unavailability of records.

The researchers concluded that motivational factors were the most important source of response error in the financial surveys. Supporting evidence included failures to report the existence of savings accounts even when the balance was fairly high, as in the study of owners of savings accounts with balances of $1000 or more. Also, many respondents simply refused to provide information on account balances. When information was provided, errors tended to be understatements, which again indicates a desire to conceal.

In the studies of debt, also, many individuals simply failed to report the debt in question, even though they likely knew the debt existed. Further support for the motivational explanation was obtained from the fact that when efforts were made to overcome respondents' resistance to disclose, as in the sealed-envelope technique, accuracy improved.

---

[9]Apparently, only 3 of the 89 interviewees were associated with accounts that were opened after January 1, 1959. Where these three cases fell in terms of response disposition was not reported.

A final note: Comparisons among the many studies of savings account owners with respect to the reporting of amounts must be made with caution since the standards for determining accuracy varied — to the exact dollar, by a specific percentage or margin, or within a given range. If a specific margin was used — for example, plus or minus $50 — errors may have been more probable for larger accounts. Other possible problems have been discussed in connection with specific studies.

Summary and Conclusions

1. Percentages of accurate responses for the 67 financial matters questions reviewed herein ranged from .4% — admittedly an extreme score — to 100%.

2. Factors discussed with respect to their potential impact on response accuracy were generally the same as those identified in the previous two chapters. In addition to those factors, the following variables emerged as potentially influencing accuracy:

   a. Question context. This refers, for example, to the impact of preceding questions on the subject's understanding of what is currently being requested.
   b. The number of topics covered in a survey, or the length of the interview/questionnaire. This relates to a respondent's ability to focus and to the subject's ability or willingness to spend sufficient time on any particular question.
   c. Interviewer's direct assistance, for example, in calculating amounts.
   d. Interviewer's prior awareness of what would constitute a truthful response.
   e. Interviewer's misinterpretation of response.

3. Factors interact to affect response accuracy.

6

Accuracy Levels in Surveys: Factors Affecting Response Accuracy — Discussion and Conclusions

Rates of Accuracy

Responses to some of the questions in the studies reviewed were highly accurate. In general, however, there was a great deal of error in these responses to survey questions. In some cases, as discussed in the text, the criterion applied may have been inaccurate or inappropriate. However, the use of inexact criteria would most likely explain only a small portion of the invalidity found.

Across and within each of the three very general question topic categories represented in the preceding chapters, there was wide variation in the percentages of accurate responses to the questions reviewed. Question topic, in and of itself, does not appear to either guarantee or discourage accurate responding.

Factors Affecting Response Accuracy

Variables Identified in This Review

In our exploration of the studies and questions included in this review, we identified 28 factors that appeared to be associated with response accuracy or inaccuracy. These factors are described in the Summary and Conclusions section of each of the three preceding chapters and are summarized in Table 6.1. These variables are further assigned to one of the three general classes of reasons for response error which constituted the framework with which we began our investigation (see Chapter 2). While many of the factors could be classified into more than one category, we attempted to choose a primary category for each variable. In certain cases, as, for example, with method, more than one classification was clearly appropriate.

Knowledge about the level of any one of these factors with respect to a particular question, however, does not necessarily allow any predictions to be made with respect to response accuracy. To illustrate this point, we will discuss several of the identified factors with respect to survey questions included in this review.

Table 6.1 Variables Affecting Response Accuracy

	General reasons for response error		
Variables affecting response accuracy	Inaccessibility of information to respondent	Problems of communication	Motivational factors
Whether respondent ever had the requested information	X		
Length of the recall period	X		
Salience of the behavior	X		
Distortions in recall caused by related experiences	X		
Memory reconstruction	X		
Social desirability/self-presentation			X
Survey method	X	X	X
Question clarity		X	
Respondent characteristics	X	X	X
Acquiescence response set			X
Interest in or commitment to survey			X
Opportunity to check records or consult with other people	X		
Question sensitivity/privacy of subject			X
Anonymity/confidentiality			X
Amount of specificity required in response	X		
Use of proxy respondents	X		

(*continues*)

In some cases, behaviors or events that would be suspected of being salient to the respondents were reported more accurately. For example, responses to questions on past voting behavior were generally not very accurate except concerning elections which may have been more salient, such as presidential elections. Similarly, in the hospitalization study which used a 1-year time frame, responses to the very salient question of whether surgery was performed were highly accurate. As additional examples, Weaver & Swanson's (1974) respondents were mostly accurate in reporting their dates of birth, as were Ball's (1967) subjects in identifying their first arrest.

Salience, however, was not necessarily associated with accuracy. For example, in Locander *et al.*'s (1976) study, response error was high for both the bankruptcy and the drunk driving questions. Also, Hyman (1944) found a substantial amount of invalidity in responses concerning recent war bond redemption.

Table 6.1 (*continued*)

Variables affecting response accuracy	General reasons for response error		
	Inaccessibility of information to respondent	Problems of communication	Motivational factors
Knowledge/suspicion that responses would be validated			X
Beliefs about the purpose of the survey			X
Setting in which survey is conducted		X	X
Question threat/fear of self-incrimination			X
Interviewer's ability to establish rapport		X	X
Time to reflect	X		
Whether question requires a yes/no response or specification of an amount or frequency	X		
Question context	X	X	
Length of survey/number of topics covered	X		X
Interviewer's assistance	X	X	X
Interviewer's awareness of "correct" response		X	X
Interviewer's misinterpretation of response		X	

In some cases, there were method effects. The best evidence is from studies by Locander *et al.* (1976), Cannell & Fowler (1963), Rogers (1976), and Lansing *et al.* (1961), where respondents were asked the same question through different approaches. In Cannell & Fowler's (1963) hospitalization study, the questionnaire seemed to be superior to the personal interview method for questions where information might be found in records, which could be consulted as respondents completed the questionnaire. For other questions, the authors believed that the interviewer's skill could assist recall. Interviewers may also help clarify the meaning of a question. For the questions on diagnosis, which many respondents probably didn't know and which might not be contained in records, and on whether surgery was performed, which was undoubtedly quite salient, method made no difference.

In Rogers' (1976) study on voting behavior, respondents were more accurate by telephone than in person. Lansing *et al.* (1961) concluded that a condition in which a sealed envelope was used to increase the perception of anonymity was superior for obtaining accurate reports concerning whether a cash loan was made.

In Locander *et al.*'s (1976) study, the methods were fairly comparable in terms of response accuracy except for the questions on the socially undesirable behaviors of drunken driving arrests and bankruptcy involvement. For those behaviors, the random response method appears to have been best. The effect of method, however, was not significant over all questions asked in this study.

The degree of threat posed by a question appears to have influenced accuracy in certain instances. For example, as might be expected, the descriptive information and recent voting behavior questions, which may be comparatively nonthreatening, tended to have fairly high percentages of accurate responses. Also, some questions which may be considered more threatening tended to have predictably low levels of accuracy. These included questions concerning savings account balances and underreporting of income on tax returns.

Counter to what might be expected based on a consideration of the amount of threat involved, however, respondents were quite accurate in responses to questions concerning current drug use, whether they had received money from welfare, and whether they had ever been ticketed or arrested by police. Ball (1967) noted that respondents may have answered his current drug use question so truthfully because he took steps to reduce the level of perceived threat.

The discussion of this selected group of factors also demonstrates the apparent lack of independence of factors in general with respect to their effects on accuracy. Interaction effects are important to consider.

To provide a framework for our discussion of the studies, we outlined three general reasons for response error (see Chapter 2). When the factors identified in the literature reviewed as potentially affecting response accuracy were classified according to these reasons, two major categories emerged (see Table 6.1). These concerned the accessibility of the information requested and motivational factors.

Motivational factors have received much attention in the literature. On the other hand, interest in accessibility, and the cognitive psychological processes involved in memory and information retrieval as they may relate to responding in surveys, is relatively recent. Many of the factors identified in our exploration of the research appear to involve these processes. Theories and research from cognitive psychology may therefore be especially useful for identifying relevant variables and assisting our understanding of factors and processes involved when individuals respond to survey questions about behavior or events in their lives. Because of its importance, we present a rather extensive review of the literature in cognitive psychology, focusing on topics that may be particularly relevant to the subject of survey response accuracy.

Cognitive Psychological Perspective

The Use of Categories
Researchers often provide categories for respondents to use in responding to survey questions. While the use of categories may be thought to aid recall, and while it certainly facilitates the summarizing of survey results, theories and research in cognitive psychology suggest that there are possible problems with the use of categories.

The numbers or choices provided may result in the anchoring effect (Tversky & Kahneman, 1974). That is, individuals' estimates are biased toward initial values. When starting points in the way of categories are provided, respondents' adjustments may be inadequate.

As another example of a possible problem, Reder (1987) reported that subjects' impressions of the questioning situation can affect the response strategy used. Perhaps when categories are provided the implicit expectation is that respondents will make estimates, as opposed to recalling exact amounts.

Additionally, subjects offered categories may assume that the correct response is represented, when in fact it may not be. This belief may create a pressure to choose, which may increase the likelihood of untruthful responses.

That this outcome is a possibility when categories are used is indirectly supported in the work of Cutler, Penrod, & Martens (1987). In their research, subjects viewed a videotaped reenactment of a crime and were later asked to make an identification of the offender from a lineup. Just half of the subjects were shown a lineup where the offender was actually present.[1] In all, however, 82% of the subjects made an identification. We can perhaps think of lineup members as being similar to categories. Cutler *et al.* (1987) concluded that the "high choosing rate may reflect a generally high a priori belief that the lineup contains the perpetrator or may indicate a judgmental strategy in which witnesses identify the lineup member who best resembles the perpetrator (Lindsay and Wells, 1985)" (p. 251).

The above finding led Cutler *et al.* (1987) to surmise that eyewitness identifications from a lineup will be *more* probable the *less* vivid the image of the perpetrator. The more vivid, the greater the necessity for a close match. If the image is less vivid, an approximation will suffice. In fact, the researchers found that subjects in poor encoding conditions made more positive identifications than subjects exposed to better encoding conditions. Yet the relationship found between choosing and identification accuracy was −.50.

Vividness of recollection may be similar to accessibility, or the availability to recall of the requested information. If so, this research on eyewitness identification suggests that the less accessible the information, the greater the likelihood that an individual will select an approximation from the categories presented, as opposed to looking for an exact match. The probability of inaccuracy is also thereby increased.

Ericsson & Simon (1980) also note that if respondents are offered an inadequate set of fixed alternatives, they may resort to "intermediate and inferential processing" (p. 222), as opposed to recalling the actual information. Although Ericsson and Simon were discussing reports of cognitive processes, the same conjecture can reasonably be made with respect to the recall of autobiographical information.

Loftus & Palmer (1974) found that the phrasing of a question about an event can affect not only responses, but also can apparently transform the memory of an event.[2] The possibility that stored information can be modified or recoded was also discussed by Tulving & Thomson (1973). Categories

---

[1] In surveys, this problem is addressed by offering respondents categories which are believed to be exhaustive.

[2] Close to 97% of a group of 63 experts on eyewitness testimony identified the phenomenon concerning the effect of question wording on responses as "'reliable enough for psychologists to present ... in courtroom testimony'" (p. 1092), indicating widespread acceptance in the scientific community (Kassin, Ellsworth, & Smith, 1989). In fact, of 21 topics evaluated by the experts in that study, the question wording topic had the highest percentage of endorsements as a "reliable enough" (p. 1093) phenomenon.

provided for respondents in surveys are a part of the phrasing of the question and as such may suggest responses and alter memories.

Response Time and Response Strategies

Response accuracy may be related to the amount of time taken to respond (Loftus, Fienberg, & Tanur, 1985). In an article concerning the cognitive processes involved in responding to survey questions calling for quantitative answers, Bradburn, Rips, & Shevell (1987) noted that:

> Increasing the amount of time for a response can affect the strategy a respondent uses, as well as the accuracy of the resulting answer (Tourangeau *et al.*, 1986; Burton & Blair, 1986). One effect of longer questions is to give people more time to recall events, thus producing better responses (Cannell *et al.*, 1977). [p. 158]

In particular, the retrieval of comparatively inaccessible information may be time consuming. Support for this possibility can be found in the description of long-term memory (LTM) offered by Ericsson & Simon (1980) in their model of human cognitive processing:

> The LTM may be pictured as an enormous collection of interrelated nodes. Nodes can be accessed either by recognitions . . . or by way of links that associate these nodes to others that have already been activated. Information accessed by association is then also represented by pointers in STM [short-term memory]. Thus, information can be brought into STM from sensory stimuli via the recognition process, or from LTM via the association process. Association processes are much slower than direct recognition processes, requiring at least several hundred milliseconds for each associative step. Associative processes may use STM to store intermediate steps. So, for example, in recalling a name that is *not immediately accessible,* a person may use a sequence of cues to find an associative path, step by step, to the sought-for name. Such processes may last *tens of seconds, or even minutes,* and may leave numerous intermediate symbols in STM, where they are temporarily available for verbal reports. [p. 224, emphases added]

Research support for the conclusion that inaccessible information takes relatively more time to retrieve may be found in the work of Baddeley, Lewis, Eldridge, & Thomson (1984). In one of their experiments, subjects were required to respond "yes" to positive instances of a previously announced category. Responses to items that represented frequently occurring instances, or what were called salient items, were made significantly more rapidly and more accurately than were responses to items representing infrequently occurring instances, a result that was consistent with prior research findings (e.g., Wilkins, 1971). In other words, the less accessible the item, the longer the response time. Further, Reiser, Black, & Abelson (1985), in discussing autobiographical experiences, concluded that, "Older memories are less accessible than more recent memories ... and ... generally take longer to retrieve" (p. 108).

We can also speculate further as to why, when respondents are asked to provide comparatively inaccessible information, accuracy would be increased if individuals were given more time to respond. An understanding of this process is important for the further development of methods and procedures to increase survey response validity.

Recall that Bradburn *et al.* (1987) stated that "Increasing the amount of time for a response can affect the strategy a respondent uses" (p. 158). Research by Reder (1987) provides evidence that individuals in fact choose response strategies and that these choices are influenced by factors both intrinsic and extrinsic to the question. Intrinsic factors include the recency or familiarity of the event in question. Extrinsic factors discussed by Reder include task requirements or instructions. In research on the recall of prose passages, Hasher & Griffin (1978) found that the procedures employed at the time of recall influenced the recall strategy used by respondents. As noted earlier in this review, Ericsson & Simon (1980) concluded that offering subjects an inadequate set of alternatives may affect the response strategy used.

For the retrieval of specific autobiographical experiences, Reder (1987) stated that respondents would need to use a "successive refinement strategy" (p. 130), as described, for example, in the model of memory organization proposed by Reiser *et al.* (1985). This memory search strategy, according to Reder, basically involves a "search for relevant contexts" (p. 130) in which to find the answer. If the successive refinement strategy was chosen,

> ... the answerer would have to predict a plausible memory location for an event that might have the relevant target features. When the features sought are not found there, a new location is tried or an assessment is made of the probability of finding the required information. [Reder, 1987, p. 130]

According to Reiser *et al.* (1985), in autobiographical retrieval, strategic processes such as inference mechanisms direct the search to and within appropriate contexts or knowledge structures. Some knowledge structures contain generalizations "that have been abstracted from individual experiences" (p. 91), while others are specific activity categories. Particular experiences are linked or associated to these knowledge structures.

It makes sense that, as compared to accessible information, a search for comparatively inaccessible information would require more in the way of time and effort. In fact, accessibility might be defined in terms of the amount of search effort or processing time required.[3] The more extensive the search, or the more inaccessible the information, the more time would be needed. However, if one of the external factors is an implicit time constraint, as might be the case with binary questions, that is, questions which call for a "yes" or "no" response, the search may be truncated.

Respondents, however, still want to provide an answer. Under pressure to quickly respond, subjects may select an ineffective strategy from the point of view of survey researchers. For example, respondents may use a purely re-constructive approach, relying heavily on such mechanisms as inference and integration, as opposed to a reproductive strategy, that is, attempting exact recall (Hasher & Griffin, 1978). In fact, in one of Reder's experiments, subjects' strategy choices were influenced by external cues in the form of instructions to use a particular response strategy, even though at times performance suffered.

Banaji & Crowder (1989) discussed the difficulty of determining whether subjects' responses to questions about past events are based on actual mem-ories of those events or on general knowledge concerning events of that type. This general knowledge was referred to as "scripts" or "generic infor-mation" (p. 1190) and is like the type of abstract information contained in the general action knowledge structures described by Reiser *et al.* (1985) or in the scripts discussed by Abelson (1981). According to Banaji and Crowder (1989):

> In Strube and Neubauer's (1988) study of memory for oral exami-
> nations, it is possible that memory for when the oral exam oc-
> curred could be as much a function of actually remembering the
> time of day as it could be the knowledge that oral examinations
> in a certain institution were usually scheduled in the morning.
> [p. 1190]

Bradburn *et al.* (1987) discussed three basic strategies or procedures that respondents apparently use to respond to requests for personal quanti-tative information—recall and count, decomposition, and the "availability bias" (p. 160). Importantly, only the recall-and-count strategy appears to ex-clusively involve an attempt to retrieve the specific information from long term memory. The other procedures described by Bradburn *et al.*

---

[3]Of course, retrieval time is at least partially dependent on the effectiveness of retrieval cues, as represented by the survey question or questions. Some cues are more useful at directing retrieval than others. Further, less effective cues add processing time (Reiser, Black, & Abelson, 1985). The importance of cues in the retrieval process is discussed more fully later in this chapter.

(1987) seem to involve, at least in part, the use of inference processes by respondents.[4]

Decomposition, for example, while apparently at least partially dependent on retrieving specific items from LTM, is a technique which may also typically include the use of inference. When asked, for example, how many times they have performed an activity over a specified period of time, respondents may first determine the rate of occurrence in a shorter time frame and then expand that rate through multiplication to cover the entire reference period.

The third technique, called the "availability bias" (Bradburn *et al.*, 1987, p. 160), relies the most heavily on inference. That is, when events are quickly recalled, respondents are likely to infer that the events occurred frequently or recently (also see Tversky & Kahneman, 1974).

According to Bradburn *et al.* (1987), while decomposition can be an effective technique to improve the accuracy of responses to questions asking for personal quantitative information, in general, inference "is at best inexact and at worst misleading" (p. 161). But if not given enough time to respond to questions calling for comparatively inaccessible information, subjects may tend to rely on these inference processes which, in fact, may demand less time and effort than reproductive strategies such as recall and count.

Evidence supports that retrieving autobiographical information from long term memory is demanding, and that respondents would choose simpler procedures if possible. In this regard, Bradburn *et al.* (1987) noted that, "Although some data suggest that no event entirely disappears from memory . . . , the effort required for retrieval can be immense, exceeding the capacity of even the most motivated respondent" (p. 158).

Bradburn *et al.* (1987) also concluded that the use of the recall-and-count strategy by respondents decreased as the length of the reference period or the frequency of occurrence increased. A similar finding was obtained in a study by Bruce and Read, as cited in Banaji & Crowder (1989), in which the subject of the study was asked to recall the frequency of a number of events that had occurred during a vacation. The subject indicated that she "tended to remember and tally the specific instances of low frequency events . . . [and] relied more on general impressions when judging the number of occurrences of higher frequency events" (p. 1189). Perhaps the use of the recall-and-count strategy decreases as processing demands increase.

---

[4]Inference processes in this context are *not* like the inference processes described by Reiser, Black, & Abelson (1985), whereby inference mechanisms guide the retrieval of particular experiences. In contrast, the inference processes described by Bradburn, Rips, & Shevell (1987) appear to be used *in place of* specific information retrieval efforts. The distinction appears to be between an inference-driven search on the one hand and an inference-based response on the other.

The retrieval of certain types of information, then, may demand a great deal of effort. Baddeley *et al.* (1984) noted that "It seems plausible to assume that the time to retrieve . . . [low-salience or low-instance frequency] items . . . [in a category-recognition task] . . . is longer, and the process of retrieval itself, more demanding" (p. 531).

Reiser *et al.* (1985) also found that the retrieval of comparatively less frequent "failure actions" (p. 103), for example, "didn't get what you asked for" (p. 103), was more difficult and took longer.

Ericsson & Simon (1980) argued that retrieving information from memory, in this case, about cognitive processes, "requires considerable time and effort, and we would claim that subjects, unless explicitly instructed to provide a relatively complete recall, would be highly unlikely to do so, *especially if other processing alternatives were available to them*" (p. 246, emphasis added). These "alternatives" may include generating answers through the use of inferences—inferences based, for example, on the vividness of recollections or on hypotheses based on self-descriptions or normative expectations. Inferences may also be based on respondents' own beliefs or naive explanations for behavior, or on their developed system of behavioral rules.

In a related vein, Tversky & Kahneman (1974) concluded that, under conditions of uncertainty, when assessing probabilities or predicting values, individuals "rely on a limited number of heuristic principles which reduce the *complex tasks* of assessing probabilities and predicting values to *simpler judgmental operations*" (p. 1124, emphases added).

Generating answers through the use of such processes as inference without directly accessing the particular items of information may not only be easier for respondents, but may, in fact, constitute a natural tendency. Research indicates that specific items of information, or experiences, are categorized or associated in LTM (Ericsson & Simon, 1980). In other words, information is not simply stored. Rather, experiences are organized, integrated, simplified, and abstracted (e.g., Nelson & Friedrich, 1980; Abelson, 1981; Reiser *et al.*, 1985).

This type of information processing makes sense when we consider *why* the information is being collected, namely to guide future activities, such as problem solving, behavior, prediction, and inference. Abstractions, generalizations, rules, and beliefs accomplish this purpose.[5] It is difficult to imagine

---

[5] A consideration of the function of memory in our lives may also help explain the finding in Tulving & Thomson's (1973) research that when cues were presented with target words, the cues later presented alone were more effective in eliciting target word responses than were target words presented alone in eliciting the cues. Subjects expected to be tested for target words in the presence of the cues. The cues, then, functioned as stimuli. In their research, therefore, the stimuli were attended to such that they controlled access to stored information, while the responses, although also attended to, did not have this control function. (*continues*)

how knowledge of discrete experiences only could act as an efficient and effective source of information for action decisions.

Consulting abstractions or generalizations, then, is more natural for respondents than retrieving information about particular experiences, which may, in fact, represent rule deviations. That cognitive processing indeed tends toward efficiency has been suggested by Abelson (1981). To consult individual items in our memory "files" takes time and effort. For questions about comparatively inaccessible information, question formats which require more than a simple "yes" or "no" response may provide respondents with more time to respond—time to use cognitive strategies which are more productive of accurate responses.

Retrieval Cues

Researchers and theorists in cognitive psychology have concluded that for the accurate retrieval of information from long-term memory, certain types of cues or probes are more effective than others (e.g., Ericsson & Simon, 1980; Bradburn *et al.*, 1987). An effective cue has been defined by Tulving & Thomson (1973) as "one whose presence facilitates recall in comparison with free or nominally noncued recall" (p. 354).

Tulving & Pearlstone (1966) found that information recall was dependent not only on the availability of the information in long-term memory, but also on retrieval cues which affect its accessibility. Thomson & Tulving (1970) concluded that the "retrieval of event information can only be effected by retrieval cues corresponding to a part of the total encoding pattern representing the perceptual cognitive registration of the occurrence of the event" (p. 261). In other words, a "target item must be encoded in some sort of reference to the cue for the cue to be effective" (Tulving & Thomson, 1973, p. 359).

Interestingly, Tulving & Thomson (1973) found that on a task calling for the recall of target words in the face of effective cues, that is, cues present at the time of encoding, subjects' performance was better than on a task calling for the recognition of these target words when they were presented with other distractor words. In the latter task, target words may have been similar to

---

(*continued*) This attention to stimuli in such a way that they can control, elicit, or release responses may be efficient and adaptive. We cannot attend to all of the features of our environment. The following comment by Markus (1980) was made in reference to our attentional processes in our social worlds, but is no doubt applicable to attention in general. "We focus on those aspects of the . . . environment that we *need* to attend to." (p. 102, emphasis added).

Brown & McNeill (1966) speculated that differences in attention may account for the fact that certain features of low-frequency words are more easily retrieved than others. They concluded that "the features favored by attention . . . appear to carry more information than the features that are not favored" (p. 325).

categories in that subjects were asked to choose a correct response from among a set of alternatives. Tulving & Thomson's (1973) research suggests that, for optimal retrieval, efforts should be focused on constructing questions that contain effective cues, as opposed to developing categories that, although relevant for data analysis, may actually decrease response accuracy.

Conclusions about the relative effectiveness of cues are often based on assumptions concerning information processing and storage and memory organization; in effect, taking advantage of the naturally occurring organization, just as we do when we develop search strategies (Reiser *et al.*, 1985). (On the other hand, research findings on the relative effectiveness of cues have also been useful in the development of theories about cognitive structures and processes.) For example, Reiser *et al.* (1985) found that specific activity cues, as opposed to general action cues, were associated with faster retrievals of autobiographical experiences. Their results also point to an "optimal level of (cue) constraint" (p. 123) in terms of specificity.

Question Context

The importance of context has also been discussed by researchers. Nelson, Bajo, & Casanueva (1985), for example, discussed the importance of "modifying contextual cues" (p. 99) in reducing interference in recall.

In an apparent reference to context, Bradburn *et al.* (1987) noted that "Questions that seek information without prior warning — including most survey questions — are especially susceptible to availability bias (Hastie and Park, 1986)" (p. 160). Bradburn *et al.* suggested that autobiographical sequences might be used to help respondents locate events in time. The authors also commented that accuracy may be improved by encouraging respondents to use the technique of decomposition "when it fails to occur naturally" (p. 160). As previously described, decomposition as a recall strategy asks for respondents to determine the rate of occurrence of a behavior over a shorter time frame than that being referred to in the survey question. Respondents then project that rate over the entire reference period.

Bekerian & Bowers (1983) suggested that "access depends on the retrieval environment emphasizing features *present at the time of original encoding* . . . , [specifically], . . . thematic information." [p. 143; emphasis added]

Bower (1981) referred to emotions as "internal contexts" (p. 136). His subjects learned word lists while they were experiencing a particular hypnotically induced emotion, either happy or sad, and then they were presented with an interfering word list learning task. Free recall of the original material was facilitated if the subjects were in the same mood at the time of retrieval as at the time of original learning. This effect was labeled mood state-dependent retrieval. In effect, "mood reinstatement" (p. 136) acted as a type of "search clue" (p. 136). Bower acknowledged, however, that mood matching is unnecessary if "adequate retrieval cues are provided" (p. 136), that is, cues directly or specifically associated with the target information. Overall, however, the findings concerning affective state-dependent recall have been mixed (Blaney, 1986). Nevertheless, there does appear to be a consensus that emotion is generally a comparatively weak, that is, indirect, cue (Bower, 1981; Blaney, 1986; Reiser et al., 1985).

Schachter (1986) cited a review by Eich (1980) that presented "experimental evidence that alcohol and other drugs can produce state-dependent memory effects in nonalcoholic volunteers" (p. 289). In this case, the context is the state of intoxication. Reinstatement of this state prompted the recall of events that occurred when the subjects were previously intoxicated.

Reiser et al. (1985) concluded that details of an experience should be remembered better if individuals first reconstruct the activity context for the experience, in other words, ask themselves what they were doing when the experience took place. Questions designed to encourage activity context reconstruction should enable, then, better and faster recall. Reiser et al. further hypothesized that once an activity context has been accessed, it should be easier for subjects to stay within that activity than to access another activity. In a related vein, Tulving & Pearlstone (1966) concluded that the recall of words from a particular category resulted in other words in that category becoming more accessible for retrieval.

The implications of this possibility for survey construction are that questions about a particular activity should be grouped and that focused surveys may produce higher levels of accuracy than omnibus-type surveys. Surveys that explore many different activities or experiences may place too many processing demands on respondents. After a time, subjects may opt for simpler strategies as opposed to direct retrieval. If so, we might find a "position order effect" on accuracy. This would be especially problematic in surveys that place their "target" questions near the end.

Summary: Factors Influencing Response Accuracy

We have identified a large number of variables that potentially affect the validity of survey responses. Many of these factors emerged from our review of the studies included in this report. Other factors were suggested by research and theories in cognitive psychology. Although typically not explicitly addressing the problem of response inaccuracy in surveys, this body of knowledge relates to the more basic concern with the processes involved in memory and information retrieval. As suggested in our review of certain specific topics, the cognitive psychological perspective promises to be a fruitful one for the identification of sources of inaccuracy and for the development of methods to increase response validity. The findings in cognitive psychology were considered in the identification of variables to include in the meta-analysis and were particularly useful in the interpretation of our findings.

Effect on Accuracy of the Incidence of Behavior Performance

Cahalan's (1968) hypothesis that inaccuracy will be decreased in cases where the incidence of performance of the behavior is high and where distortions tend to be overstatements was supported by the data. Not supported is the implication that highly inaccurate responses will be obtained to questions about socially desirable behavior when they are directed to groups within which the behavior has a low incidence of performance.

For example, Weiss (1968) found that her subjects were quite accurate (82%) in their responses to a voting question, even though the incidence of actual voting was low (29%). Again, distortions were overwhelmingly false claims (16% versus 2% understatements). Also, in Katosh & Traugott's (1981) study on voting behavior in the 1976 and 1978 elections, the percentages of accurate responses were similar (87% versus 86%), even though the turnout rates were quite different (61% versus 43%).

Cahalan's hypothesis also suggests that high accuracy will result when the incidence of performance is low and distortions tend to be understatements. Support for this expectation was found in some of the findings in the studies reviewed, for example, in Clark & Tifft's (1966) study of deviant and sexual behavior.

Areas for Further Exploration

As previously stated, one of our major goals in this work was to determine the level of accuracy in responses to survey questions about behavior and personal characteristics. Having reviewed a large number of studies which examined the accuracy of individuals' responses, we concluded that there appears to be a high level of inaccuracy in survey responses.

What is the effect of this inaccuracy in survey responses on the conclusions researchers reach? In Chapter 7, we explore this question by comparing results based on data obtained from self-reports with results based on data obtained from records or other sources and used as criteria in the investigations reviewed in this report.

Another issue raised in the course of our exploration is whether inaccuracy is respondent related or item specific. Certain respondents may tend to be untruthful, irrespective of the question posed. On the other hand, untruthfulness may be more closely associated or dependent on particular item or question characteristics. This issue is also addressed in Chapter 7.

Our second major goal in this investigation was to identify and systematically evaluate factors associated with response accuracy. From our review of the studies included in this report, a large number of factors emerged as potentially affecting response validity. In addition, from the literature in cognitive psychology, we identified a number of other variables that may be important to consider in this regard.

A systematic, quantitative assessment of our data in the form of a meta-analysis is described in detail in Part IV. Through this procedure, we sought to determine the relative influence on accuracy of a number of variables and to identify dominant factors. Further, in our review we found that variables appear to interact in terms of their effects on accuracy. Variable interactions, therefore, were also included for assessment in the meta-analysis.

Part III

Other Issues in Survey Research

7

Implications and Patterns of Inaccuracy

Consequences of Using Self-Report versus Actual Data

One way to evaluate the effect of response error on research conclusions is to compare aggregate level self-report data with actual values, specifically the percentages of respondents answering the questions who are identified as involved, as opposed to the percentages of respondents that actually were involved in the subject in question. Comparisons of aggregate level self-report data with actual values for all questions where this information was available in the studies reviewed in this report are presented in Table 7.1. Of 79 comparisons, only 4 are identical. However, small deviations may be acceptable.

The similarity of the reported to the actual percentages was assessed in two ways. First, the range for the ratios of the reported to the actual percentages is from .25 for one of the questions on income tax reporting to 11.50 for the question on the display of a poster, an extreme example. Because the ratios for reverse record check studies will never be greater than 1, for the purpose of comparability, for all of the questions we calculated the absolute difference between a perfect match, represented by a ratio of 1.00, and the obtained ratio, a measure that we refer to as the absolute error score. These scores range from 0 to 1050.

The percentages of cases that fall into particular absolute error score intervals are presented in Fig. 7.1. If an absolute error score of 10 or less is considered to be a satisfactory interval for finding aggregate reported estimates similar to the actual, then in only 19% ($N = 15$) of the cases can the reported and actual values be considered similar. Another 18% ($N = 14$) fall just outside this interval, but 63% ($N = 50$) of the cases are extremely

Table 7.1 Actual versus Self-Reported Data: Percentage of Sample Involved

| | | | Findings Based On | | | | | | 95% Confidence interval | |
| | | Number asked | Self-report data (%) | | | Actual data (%) | Ratio of reported to actual | Absolute error score | | |
Study	Information requested		Accurate[a]	+	Over[b]				Low (%) −	High (%)[c]
Reports of descriptive information										
Cahalan (1968);	Possession of driver's license	920	44	+	10 = 54	46	1.17	17	50.8 −	57.2*
Parry & Crossley (1950); Crossley & Fink (1951)	Possession of a valid library card	902	11.2	+	9.2 = 20.4	13.3	1.53	53	17.8 −	23.0*
	Automobile ownership	892	60.9	+	3.1 = 64	60.9	1.05	5	60.9 −	67.2
	Home ownership	920	53	+	3 = 56	54	1.04	4	52.8 −	59.2
	Telephone in household	920	84	+	1 = 85	85	1.00	0	82.7 −	87.3
Reports of various events and behaviors										
Weiss (1968)	Child's failure of a subject on his last report card	416	27.5	+	10 = 37.5	54.6	.69	31	32.8 −	42.2*
	Child's ever being left back to repeat a grade in school	400	30.2	+	12 = 42.2	39.7	1.06	6	37.4 −	47.0
Hyman (1944)	Whether received government posters	790	86.[a]			100	.86	14	83.6 −	88.4*
	Whether received a specific poster known to have been mailed about 10 days earlier	679	32.5			100	.33	67	29.0 −	36.0*
	Whether poster was put on display	221	4	+	42 = 46	4	11.50	1050	39.4 −	52.6*
Reports of attendance and absenteeism										
Hyman (1944)	Whether absent recently	158	96.2			100	.96	4	93.2 −	99.2*
	Whether absent in the last couple of months	134	66.4			100	.66	34	58.4 −	74.4*
Gray (1955)	Whether sick leave taken in the period July–November 15	433	47.1	+	3 = 50.1	52.7	.95	5	45.4 −	54.8

118

Reports of cigarette smoking

Study	Item													
Bauman et al. (1982)	Recency of smoking cigarettes (Group I)	43	4.7	+	0	=	4.7	4.7	1.00	0	0.0	–	15.0
	Recency of smoking cigarettes (Group II)	39	7.7	+	0	=	7.7	7.7	1.00	0	2.0	–	21.0

Reports of voting behavior

Clausen (1968)	Whether voted for president on November 3, 1964	1110	74.5	+	2.3	=	76.8	75.1	1.02	2	74.3	–	79.3
Freeman (1953)	Whether voted in recent (1950) election	374	56.2	+	15.2	=	71.4	58.3	1.22	22	66.8	–	76.0*
Miller (1952)	Whether voted in recent (1950) congressional elections	204	53.9	+	10.8	=	64.7	53.9	1.20	20	58.1	–	71.3*
Katosh & Traugott (1981)	1978 registration status	2230	60.6	+	12.3	=	72.9	62.7	1.16	16	71.1	–	74.7*
	1978 voting behavior	2222	41.9	+	12.8	=	54.7	43.2	1.27	27	52.6	–	56.8*
	1976 registration status	2344	65.8	+	12.3	=	78.1	69	1.13	13	76.4	–	79.8*
	1976 voting behavior	2329	59.7	+	12.3	=	72	60.8	1.18	18	70.2	–	73.8*
Cahalan (1968); Parry & Crossley (1950); Crossley & Fink (1951)	Whether voted in 1948 presidential election	920	60	+	13	=	73	61	1.20	20	70.1	–	75.9*
	Whether voted in September, 1948 primary election	856	25.8	+	22.5	=	48.3	29	1.67	67	45.0	–	51.7*
	Whether voted in 1947 City Charter election	828	18.8	+	31.2	=	50	21.1	2.37	137	46.6	–	53.4*
	Whether voted in May, 1947 mayoral election	911	35.3	+	28.3	=	63.6	36.3	1.75	75	60.5	–	66.7*
	Whether voted in November, 1946 congressional election	828	30	+	21.1	=	51.1	32.2	1.59	59	47.7	–	54.5*
	Whether voted in 1944 presidential election	902	36.7	+	23.5	=	60.2	38.8	1.55	55	57.0	–	63.4*
Tittle & Hill (1967)	Voting behavior in a student election 1 week prior	296	51	+	9.5	=	60.5	51	1.19	19	54.9	–	66.1*

(continues)

Table 7.1 (*continued*)

Study	Information requested	Number asked	Self-report data (%) Accurate[a]	+	Over[b]	=	Actual data (%)	Ratio of reported to actual	Absolute error score	95% Confidence interval Low (%)	–	High (%)[c]
Rogers (1976)	Whether voted in the 1973 New York City mayoral election (telephone)	81	44	+	20	= 64	45	1.42	42	53.5	–	74.5*
	Whether voted in the 1973 New York City mayoral election (face to face)	90	37	+	26	= 63	41	1.54	54	53.0	–	73.0*
Reports of alcohol-related behavior												
Locander et al. (1976)	Whether charged with drunken driving in the last 12 months (face to face)	30	53				100	.53	47	35.1	–	70.9*
	Whether charged with drunken driving in the last 12 months (telephone)	46	54				100	.54	46	39.6	–	68.4*
	Whether charged with drunken driving in the last 12 months (questionnaire)	28	46				100	.46	54	27.5	–	64.5*
	Whether charged with drunken driving in the last 12 months (random response)	33	65				100	.65	35	48.7	–	81.3*
Sobell et al. (1974)	Ever been imprisoned in state or federal penitentiary	11	63.6				100	.64	36	31.0	–	90.0*
	Whether currently on formal probation	13	53.8				100	.54	46	25.0	–	82.0*
Reports of deviant behavior												
Ball (1967)	Drug use at time of interview	25	20	+	0	= 20	28	.71	29	4.3	–	35.7

Study	Item	N	%					%	ratio	n	%		%
Hardt & Peterson-Hardt (1977)	Ever been ticketed or arrested by police	862	15.5	+	6.5	=	22	20.1	1.09	9	19.2	–	24.8
Voss (1963)	Whether committed delinquent acts	52	98.1					100	.98	2	92.0	–	100.0
Robins (1966)	Ever been arrested	164	59					100	.59	41	51.5	–	66.5*
	Ever served time	83	71					100	.71	29	61.2	–	80.8*
Reports of sexual behavior													
Udry & Morris (1967)	Whether had coitus within the past 24 hours	15	80					100	.80	20	52.0	–	96.0*
Reports of financial matters													
Hessing et al. (1988)	Did you, when filing your 1981 tax return, underreport your income or report unwarranted deductions? (Sample I)	71	25.4					100	.25	75	15.3	–	35.5*
	Did you, when filing your 1982 tax return, underreport your income or report unwarranted deductions? (Sample I)	71	28.2					100	.28	72	17.7	–	38.7*
	Did you, when filing your 1981 tax return, underreport your income or report unwarranted deductions. (Sample II)	84	76.2[a]					100	.76	24	67.1	–	85.3*
	Did you, when filing your 1982 tax return, underreport your income or report unwarranted deductions? (Sample II)	84	79.8					100	.80	20	71.2	–	88.4*
Cahalan (1968); Parry & Crossley (1950); Crossley & Fink (1951)	Whether contributed or pledged money to Community Chest in Fall, 1948 drive	828	27.8	+	37.8	=	65.6	27.8	2.36	136	62.4	–	68.8*
Locander et al. (1976)	Ever involved in bankruptcy (face to face)	38	68					100	.68	32	53.2	–	82.8*

(continues)

Table 7.1 (*continued*)

Study	Information requested	Number asked	Self-report data (%) Accurate[a]	+	Over[b]	=	Actual data (%)	Ratio of reported to actual	Absolute error score	Low (%)	–	High (%)[c]
										95% Confidence interval		
	Ever involved in bankruptcy (telephone)	41	71				100	.71	29	57.1	–	84.9*
	Ever involved in bankruptcy (questionnaire)	31	68				100	.68	32	51.6	–	84.4*
	Ever involved in bankruptcy (random response)	26	100				100	1.00	0	88.8	–	100.0
Weiss (1968)	Whether received money from welfare	680	94.3	+	0	= 94.3	96.2	.98	2	92.6	–	96.0*
Ferber et al. (1969a)	Savings account ownership	777	54.2				100	.54	46	50.7	–	57.7*
Ferber et al. (1969b)	Common stock ownership	426	70.2				100	.70	30	65.9	–	74.5*
Maynes (1965)	Savings account ownership	2485	95				100	.95	5	94.1	–	95.9*
David (1962)	Whether received public assistance income in 1959	46	93.5				100	.94	6	83.0	–	98.0*
Hyman (1944)	Whether redeemed war bonds	243	82.7				100	.83	17	77.9	–	87.5*
Hardin & Hershey (1960)	Any change in amount of pay in the past 6 months (Survey I)	241	35	+	9	= 44	58	.76	24	37.7	–	50.3*
	Any change in amount of pay in the past 6 months (Survey II)	260	39	+	6	= 45	58	.78	22	39.0	–	51.1*
Lansing et al. (1961)												
Study I	Existence of savings account	77	76.6				100	.77	23	67.1	–	86.1*
Study III	Car loan taken: Condition A	23	73.9				100	.74	26	56.0	–	91.8*
	Car loan taken: Condition B	27	63				100	.63	37	44.8	–	81.2*
	Car loan taken: Condition C	15	40				100	.40	60	16.0	–	68.0*
	Car loan taken: Condition D	14	64.3				100	.64	36	35.0	–	89.0*

Study									
Study IV	Whether new car purchase debt was incurred	33	75.8	100	.76	24	61.2	—	90.4*
Study V	Existence of account: Method A	63	78	100	.78	22	67.8	—	88.2*
	Existence of account: Method B	46	72	100	.72	28	59.0	—	85.0*
	Existence of account 6 months ago	102	74	100	.74	26	65.5	—	82.5*
	Existence of account 1 year ago	86	74	100	.74	26	64.7	—	83.3*
	Existence of account in Fall, 1958	80	86.3	100	.86	14	78.8	—	93.8*
	Existence of account in Spring, 1959	78	84.6	100	.85	15	76.6	—	92.6*
Study VI	Whether made the cash loan: Condition A	30	30	100	.30	70	13.6	—	46.4*
	Whether made the cash loan: Condition B	34	38	100	.38	62	21.7	—	54.3*
	Whether made the cash loan: Condition C	30	50	100	.50	50	32.1	—	67.9*
Study VII	Whether account existed: Condition A	26	76	100	.76	24	59.6	—	92.4*
	Whether account existed: Condition B	25	70	100	.70	30	52.0	—	88.0*
	Whether account existed: Condition C	21	82	100	.82	18	65.6	—	98.4*
	Whether account existed: Condition D	17	68	100	.68	32	43.0	—	89.0*

*True mean not included.

[a]Accurate statements.

[b]Overstatements.

[c]The formula generally used was $\pi = P \pm 1.96\,[P(1 - P)/n]^{1/2}$. However, if N was greater than 20 but less than 60 and the proportion was equal to or less than 10 or greater than 90, or if N was less than 20, then the 95% confidence interval was estimated by reference to Figure 8.5, p. 225 in Wonnacott & Wonnacott (1977).

[d]No possibility for overstatements in reverse record check studies, because all individuals included in these studies performed the behavior or possessed a certain characteristic.

[e]For this and the following question, represents the percentage who correctly *denied* the behavior. In this table and in Figure 7.1, these two questions are categorized as reverse record check sample questions.

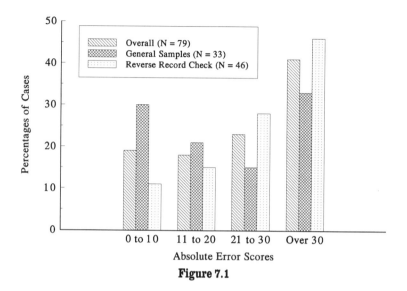

Figure 7.1

inaccurate. The distribution of absolute error scores among the topic categories reveals that both small and extremely large scores can be found in almost all question categories.

The amount of error in reverse record check studies may not be directly comparable to the amount of error in studies using general samples.[1] Also, compensating errors which can contribute to the validity of an aggregate level comparison are not possible in reverse record check studies. Therefore, error scores from the two types of studies are presented separately in Fig. 7.1. Excluding the cases that fall into the very broad "greater than 30" interval, it is apparent that as error scores increase, the percentages of cases falling into particular intervals declines for general samples and increases for reverse record check samples.

Even though 10 of these comparisons for general samples appear to be satisfactory in an aggregate sense, any individual-level analyses of the self-report data may still be problematic because of compensating errors. In one case, individuals that should have been included in the identified category were not; in another, individuals that should not have been included were; and in six cases, both types of errors occurred.

Because of the possibility of compensating errors in the data, an acceptable aggregate-level comparison is not necessarily associated with high individual-

---

[1] See discussion in Chapter 2.

level accuracy. To test the relationship between aggregate and individual-level validity for the 10 questions using general samples where the aggregate-level comparison was satisfactory (absolute error score of 10 or less), a Pearson correlation coefficient was computed between the absolute error scores resulting from the comparisons of self-report with actual data, and the corresponding overall levels of respondent accuracy. The significant negative correlation obtained ($r = -.671$, $df = 8$, $p < .05$) indicates that for these questions, high aggregate-level validity, or low error, and high individual-level accuracy tend to be related. This finding was supported by the significant negative Pearson correlation coefficient obtained when the relationship between aggregate and individual-level validity was assessed for all general sample questions ($r = -.744$, $df = 28$, $p < .001$).[2]

In the second approach, 95% confidence intervals were estimated for the 79 reported proportions (see Table 7.1). Overall, in just 12 of the cases, or 15%, the true proportion was included. For those questions in which a general sample was used, the true proportion was included in 10 of the 33, or in about 30% of those cases; for reverse record check sample questions, the true proportion was included in 2 of the 46, or in about 4% of those cases. Instances where the true proportion was *excluded* are distributed among almost all types of questions, including the descriptive information category. Because of the small number of questions in some categories, it is not possible to draw any firm conclusions. Evidence from the voting and financial questions, however — bearing in mind that financial data is almost exclusively from reverse record check studies — suggests that actual proportions will almost *never* be included within 95% confidence intervals estimated from reported data.

The data in Table 7.1 provided an opportunity to further explore the relationship between the incidence of behavioral performance and accuracy that we discussed using the data from the studies by Cahalan (1968) and Clark & Tifft (1966) (see Tables 3.7, 4.3, and 4.5). For Cahalan's socially approved behavior items, there was a significant positive association between the incidence of performance and the overall level of accuracy. In contrast, for the negative behavior items included in Clark and Tifft's study, increases in the

---

[2]Excluding Hyman's (1944) poster display question, and Cahalan's (1968) City Charter election voting and contributions to Community Chest questions, where the absolute error scores were extreme (1050, 137, and 136, respectively). For all 33 general sample questions, $r = -.504$, $df = 31$, $p < .01$. Excluding only Hyman's question, $r = -.812$, $df = 30$, $p < .001$.

Each question included in all of these analyses was weighted by the number of respondents associated with that question. The formula used to compute the weights is presented in Chapter 8.

incidence of performance were associated with increasingly low accuracy levels in reports of performance frequency.

The relationship between incidence of performance and absolute error in the comparison of actual and reported data was examined for the 22 socially desirable items for general samples.[3] It was expected that a high incidence of performance would be associated with a decreased number of overstatements, and consequently with a low absolute error score. As predicted, a significant negative Pearson correlation coefficient resulted ($r = -.835$, $df = 20, p < .001$).[4]

Only eight of the items for general samples concerned socially disapproved behaviors. For these items, although counter to expectations, the Pearson correlation coefficient was negative ($r = -.185$, $df = 6, p > .50$); it was also insignificant, indicating little association between performance and error.[5] Because of the small number of cases examined, this finding may be misleading.[6]

Inaccuracy: Respondent Characteristic or Item Dependent

One of the questions raised in our review of the primary studies was whether the tendency to be untruthful in a survey is a relatively enduring personal characteristic or behavior, as opposed to a response to specific item content or to an item in a particular context. Data from the studies by Tittle & Hill (1967), Weiss (1968), Hardin & Hershey (1960), and Weaver & Swanson (1974) support the latter conclusion.

Clancy _et al._ (1979) found that respondents who falsely claimed to have read one type of reading material were also likely to falsely claim readership of other types. Also, Hardt & Peterson-Hardt (1977), in examining the internal consistency or reliability of the responses obtained in the self-report scale

---

[3]Excluding Hyman's (1944) poster display question and Cahalan's (1968) city charter election voting and contributions to Community Chest questions, where the absolute error scores were extreme (1050, 137, and 136, respectively).

[4]For all 25 general sample questions involving socially approved behaviors, $r = -.498$, $df = 23, p < .01$. Excluding only Hyman's (1944) question, $r = -.787$, $df = 22, p < .001$. All analyses were weighted (see footnote 2 in this chapter).

[5]This analysis was weighted (see footnote 2 in this chapter).

[6]In many of the studies reviewed, the researchers attempted other types of comparisons or analyses to evaluate the consequences of using reported as opposed to actual data. In other cases, we were able to evaluate the data presented from this perspective. Although comparisons were favorable in many cases, in others, serious errors would have resulted if self-report data had been used as the basis for estimates. Information on these comparisons is available from the principal author.

used in their study, found 98% consistency in replies to two logically interrelated items, appearing about seven items apart.

The above findings may be viewed as supporting the conclusion that the tendency to report inaccurately is a respondent characteristic. Respondents, however, may have been reacting to the similar content of the two items in each study. Those respondents who were able or inclined to report accurately to questions concerning particular topics did so.

Lansing *et al.* (1961, Study V) presented data comparing the responses of interviewees to questions about their savings accounts asked in two surveys conducted approximately 6 months apart. To facilitate analysis, three categories were used to classify responses: (1) failed to report account or balance, (2) acknowledged account but reported balance was inaccurate, and (3) correctly reported the existence of account and balance (see Table 7.2).

Responses in the first survey were significantly associated with responses in the second survey ($X^2 = 55.23$, $df = 4$, $p < .001$, $v = .595$). The authors (Lansing *et al.*, 1961) commented, however, that many individuals differed in their reports from one occasion to the next:

> In other words an individual who reports accurately on one occasion probably will do so again, but one cannot have complete confidence that this will be true. This result, combined with the evidence that many respondents compromised and reported partial

Table 7.2 Relationship between Fall and Spring Reports of Savings Accounts and Balances: Distribution of Interviews

Report of account balance in spring survey	Report of account balance in fall survey			
	Failed to report account and/or balance	Inaccurate balance report[a]	Accurate balance report	Total number
Failed to report account and/or balance	24	1	3	28
Inaccurate balance report	4	12	4	20
Accurate balance report	3	6	21	30
Total number	31	19	28	78[b]

Source: Data from Lansing *et al.* (1961, Study V).

Notes: $X^2 = 55.23$, $df = 4$, $p < .001$; Cramer's V = .595.

[a]Includes both over- and underreports.

[b]"Excludes 29 respondents who were not reinterviewed in the Spring and 2 respondents whose accounts were not open on the specified date in Spring, 1959" (Lansing *et al.*, 1961, p. 89).

information about savings accounts, suggests that it would not be easy to divide respondents into two groups: accurate reporters and inaccurate reporters. [p. 90]

Lansing *et al.*s (1961, Study V) findings suggest that inaccurate reporting may be neither a response tendency nor a response to specific item content. Rather, factors peculiar to each interview situation, such as context and interviewer's expertise, may encourage accurate or inaccurate responding. Further, these factors differentially affect respondents. This conclusion is supported by Hardin & Hershey's (1960) finding of no significant relationship between the accuracy of reports of pay changes in two surveys conducted approximately 6 months apart (see Table 7.3).

Other evidence on this subject is provided by studies where the accuracy of individuals over two or more questions was assessed. If certain individuals tend to be generally untruthful, then the percentage of inaccurate respondents over two or more survey questions should not be very different from the percentages of incorrect respondents to the individual questions. On the other hand, if inaccuracy is item specific, then more respondents would be added to the inaccurate subjects pool as more questions are considered; the overall percentage of accurate respondents would then be *lower* than the percentages for individual questions. Data from the studies by Hagburg (1968) and Cahalan (1968) fit the latter circumstance, while the findings of Hessing *et al.* (1988) are consistent with the former (see Table 7.4). In

Table 7.3   Relationship between the Accuracy of Reports of Pay Changes in Two Surveys Conducted Approximately 6 Months Apart: Distribution of Interviews

Report of pay change in first survey	Report of pay change in second survey		
	Accurate	Inaccurate[a]	Total
Accurate	115	31	146
Inaccurate	47	18	65
Total	162	49	211[b]

Source: Data from Hardin & Hershey (1960).

Notes: $X^2 = 1.05$, *df* $= 1$, $p = .305$; Cramer's V $= .071$.
[a]Includes both over- and understatements.
[b]Represents the number of respondents for whom data was available for both surveys.

Table 7.4 A Comparison between the Percentages of Inaccurate Respondents to Individual Questions and the Percentages for Two or More Questions Considered Together

Study	Findings		
	Information requested	% Accurate	
Hagburg (1968)	How many Union Leadership Program classes attended:		
	The first eight weeks of this year?	53	
	The second eight weeks of this year?	48	
	Total, both questions	36	
Cahalan (1968); Parry & Crossley (1950); Crossley & Fink (1951)	Whether voted in:		
	1948 presidential election	86	
	1948 primary election	74.2	
	1947 City Charter election	66.7	
	1947 mayoral election	70.7	
	1946 congressional election	76.7	
	1944 presidential election	74.5	
	Total, six elections	41.8	
Hessing *et al.* (1988)		Sample I:	Sample II:
	Did you, when filing your 1981 tax return, underreport your income or report unwarranted deductions?	25.4	76.2
	Did you, when filing your 1982 tax return, underreport your income or report unwarranted deductions?	28.2	79.8
	Total, both questions	28	80

addition, Hessing *et al.* found a correlation of .81 ($p < .001$) between responses to the two items.

Implications and Patterns of Inaccuracy: Summary and Conclusions

Research conclusions based on self-reports were compared with actual data, with a majority of the comparisons indicating high levels of inaccuracy. When 95% confidence intervals were estimated from reported data, actual proportions were rarely included. Further, for general samples, even when aggregate-level comparisons were satisfactory, the presence of errors in the data in the form of understatements and overstatements would make any attempt to categorize individuals problematic. Our finding that aggregate-level validity and individual-level accuracy tend to be related indicates that, in general, these type errors cannot compensate for basic response invalidity.

It may not be possible to specify in advance the absolute level of accuracy desirable in a survey, as this might depend on the purpose of the survey and the subject of the investigation (Mauldin & Marks, 1950). For example, a socially undesirable behavior may be performed by only a small percentage of the population, say 6%. In a general random sample, the 94% who do not perform the behavior will probably mainly provide truthful denials. A large proportion of those who do practice the behavior, however perhaps as high as 50%, may deny it. The accuracy level of the survey would then be 97%. Yet the conclusion draw, that the behavior is performed by 3% of the population, would be a serious underestimate.

Concerning the question of whether inaccurate responding is a response tendency or personal characteristic as opposed to a behavior associated with particular item content, our data are only suggestive. Information that could be used to address this issue was presented in just a small number of the studies reviewed. Further, the items examined in each study were mainly either alike or highly similar in content, making it difficult to separate respondent behavior from item effects.

The evidence available, however, suggests that inaccurate reporting is not a response tendency or a predisposition to be untruthful. Individuals who are truthful on one occasion or in response to particular questions may not be truthful at other times or to other questions. The subject of the question, the item context, or other factors in the situation, such as interviewer expertise, may all contribute to a respondent's ability or inclination to respond truthfully. Further, the same set of conditions may differentially affect respondents, encouraging truthfulness from one and inaccurate reporting from another.

The possibility that individuals may respond differently to the same item content or characteristics or survey situation does not necessarily suggest that any endeavor to create conditions leading to high levels of response accuracy would be futile. Some of these differences in response across individuals may be attributable to differences in interviewers' style or training. Even within the same survey, there are often multiple interviewers. This possibility underscores the importance of uniformity in survey administration.

That individuals may respond differently to identical survey situations indicates that the attempt to identify factors associated with accuracy is more precisely an attempt to identify optimal item or survey characteristics, in the form of levels or combinations of variables, such that the highest possible levels of response accuracy are encouraged or facilitated for the largest number of respondents. In fact, many of the questions included in this interview achieved exactly this outcome.

In the next section of this book, we present our meta-analysis within which we identify and assess a set of variables with respect to their association with response validity.

Part IV
Meta-Analysis of Survey Responses

with Kent W. Smith

8

Meta-Analysis: Identification of Variables — Formation of Question Subsets

Introduction

In the qualitative review of percentage accurate responses to the questions from the studies included in this report, a large number of variables were identified that appeared to be related to response accuracy (especially see Chapter 6). To further our understanding of these and other variables discussed in the survey research literature, and to more precisely evaluate both their association with response accuracy and their interrelationships, a quantitative or meta-analysis was also undertaken.

As defined by Glass (1976), meta-analysis is "the statistical analysis of a large collection of analysis results from individual studies for the purpose of integrating the findings" (p. 3). This approach was selected to summarize the large amount of information gleaned from the studies reviewed and to assist our understanding of the factors associated with the wide variation in the results obtained from these studies. Further, we hoped to identify the most effective combination of variables and the optimal levels of particular variables for obtaining valid survey responses. This quantitative analysis may also be useful for making estimates concerning the probable level of accuracy of responses to questions in the absence of validating data and for guiding future survey question design efforts. The particular statistical procedure that we decided to use was regression analysis.

The process of designing, executing, and interpreting the meta-analysis or, to be exact, the meta-analyses, is described in this and in the next three chapters. In this chapter, we describe and discuss the item selection process, the variables that were identified for potential inclusion, the rationale for the separate analyses of three question subsets, and the particular variables included in each of the three analyses. The meta-analyses results are presented and briefly discussed in Chapter 9. Chapter 10 contains a detailed discussion and integration of our findings from the meta-analyses. Finally, an overall summary and our conclusions are presented in Chapter 11.

Item Selection

Of the 258 questions discussed in this review, 245 were selected for inclusion in the meta-analysis. Clancy *et al.'s* (1979) three questions on magazine readership, Cahalan's (1968) question on registration and voting in Denver 1943–1948, and King *et al.'s* (1981) question on voting in three recent school finance elections were excluded because the percentages of accuracy for these questions actually represent accuracy across more than one question and are not directly comparable to the percentage accuracy figures for the other questions. Finally, in Lansing *et al.'s* (1961) studies, four questions each from Study V and Study VI were excluded because accuracy was assessed after responses were combined across different survey methods or conditions. Therefore, any evaluation of particular method or condition effects on accuracy was not possible.

Apart from these few omitted items, the questions included in the analysis represent to the best of our knowledge the entire sample of questions from studies found in the literature during the approximate 40-year period covered in our search, where an external criterion, as defined in this report, was used to determine response validity.[1] Also, it appears that these published studies are a faithful representation of research efforts in this area in general and, as such, constitute an unbiased sample (see Rosenthal, 1978). That is, these published studies do not support a particular hypothesis concerning survey response accuracy. Rather, many of the studies were explicitly exploratory (e.g., Ball, 1967; Ito, 1963; Hardin & Hershey, 1960; Clark & Tifft, 1966; Udry & Morris, 1967; and Parry & Crossley, 1950). Further, the obtained percentage accuracy figures covered a wide range, from .4% to 100%.

Identification of Variables

Dependent Variable

The dependent variable in the meta-analysis was the percentage of truthful responses to each question.[2]

---

[1] See Chapter 1.

[2] The percentage of accurate responses to Maynes's (1965) question concerning an October, 1958 savings account balance was not reported. Therefore, this question was excluded from any analysis where the dependent variable was percentage of accurate responses.

Independent Variables

As previously noted, numerous potential independent variables we.. uis-
cussed in the qualitative report. Others have been identified in survey research literature. However, there are two reasons why it was frequently either
not possible or not feasible to obtain values for many of these variables for
every question.

First, the type of information and the amount of detail provided in the
various studies varied widely. For example, the exact question used was
frequently not stated. Even rarer was the presentation of the entire instrument used. Therefore, factors such as the degree of question clarity and
question context could not be coded for every question. As another example,
whether guarantees of anonymity or confidentiality were given to respondents was frequently not explicitly reported.

Second, the interrelationships among variables made it difficult to code
them separately. For example, whether a standard for accuracy used in
one question would be considered comparatively strict or lenient seemed
to be at least partially dependent on the length of the recall period involved, and also on the characteristics of the individuals included in the
sample.

We concluded that the influence of a large number of the identified factors
could be captured with reference to two underlying dimensions or characteristics, namely sensitivity and accessibility (see Table 8.1). This collapsing into
two main dimensions had three major benefits. First, the effects of significant
variables along these dimensions could be retained in the analysis, even if
information on these variables was missing in some studies. Second, with
only two dimensions rather than many closely related variables, we could
more readily analyze the interrelationships of these dimensions and the other
factors affecting response accuracy. Third was the related benefit that collapsing into two dimensions permitted more parsimonious explanations of how
various factors may affect response accuracy.

In addition to sensitivity and accessibility, other independent variables in
the meta-analysis were study date, response type, method, socially desirable
response direction, prevalence, and question type. The rest of this section
describes these independent variables and the procedures we used for assigning their values.

Sensitivity and Accessibility

Each of the 245 questions was assigned a sensitivity and accessibility score
based on the ratings of a panel of informed raters. To avoid the subjectivity
of any individual judgment concerning an item's sensitivity or the accessibility of the requested information to the respondent, five persons rated the

**Table 8.1 Variables Affecting Response Accuracy and
Their Associated Dimensions**

Underlying dimension	Identified variables
Accessibility	Length of recall period
	Salience of event
	Possession of requested information
	Survey method
	Selection of respondent (e.g., self versus proxy)
	Response type: binary or amount
	Standards for accuracy (e.g., exact numbers versus ranges)
	Question clarity and complexity
	Question context
	Present reality versus past behavior
	Opportunity to consult records or others
	Nature of the sample
Sensitivity	Question content or question type
	Survey method
	Question context
	Motivation to conceal or distort (e.g., social desirability, possibility of self-incrimination)
	Anonymity and confidentiality
	Motivation to be truthful (e.g., perceptions of the verifiability of information provided)
	Commitment to the study (e.g., payment for participation)
	Nature of the sample

questions on these two dimensions. All of the raters were involved in research projects at the American Bar Foundation and included the writers; a project director and an assistant project director, both of whom were familiar with research methodology and survey accuracy issues; and an administrative assistant who had only recently joined the organization and was new to the field of social science research.

Each rater was given rating sheets listing the 245 questions and the names of the respective researchers. A guide to the rating categories to be used was also provided (see Table 8.2). Every item was to be assigned two ratings from 0 to +6, representing the rater's perceptions concerning the sensitivity of the item for the respondents in the particular study and the accessibility to the respondents of the requested information. For sensitivity, "0" stood for "not at all sensitive, threatening," while "+6" meant "highly sensitive, threatening." For accessibility, "0" represented "very inaccessible, difficult to remember," and "+6" signified "accessible, easy to recall."

**Table 8.2   Guide for Scales Used to Rate Question Sensitivity
and Question Accessibility**

Factor	Rating scale						

Sensitivity
Question content, subject matter
Motives to distort (concerns
   with status, self-esteem,
   self-presentation; perceived
   social desirability of
   response)
Method
Anonymity, confidentiality
Question context
	Not at all
	sensitive or
	threatening
	0 +1
		+2	+3	+4	Highly
					sensitive,
					threatening
					+5 +6		

Accessibility
Question context
Present reality versus past behavior,
   possibility of distortion
Time frame: memory and saliency
Method
Likelihood that respondent has
   or ever had information: self
   versus proxy respondents,
   type of information
   requested
	Very
	inaccessible,
	difficult to
	remember
	0 +1
		+2	+3	+4	Accessible,
					easy to
					recall
					+5 +6		

The raters met for three lengthy meetings during which one of the writers, Wentland, presented detailed descriptions of the available information about the samples, research conditions and designs, and questions for each study. The other raters were not told what the percentages of accurate responses were, so their ratings were independent of the study results. The rationale for our decision to provide raters with detailed descriptions of the studies and questions is as follows.

As a pilot test, we started out presenting a minimum of details to certain individuals not associated with our project, none of whom eventually served as a coder. These individuals demanded more information, feeling that they could best make a judgment about accessibility and sensitivity only if they had as many facts as possible. The raters in our study felt, and we agreed, that the best judgments could be made when as much information about the study as possible was made available, apart from the level of accuracy obtained. This would include information about the method used, since method could impact sensitivity and accessibility. Global judgments about accessibility and sensitivity had to be based on many characteristics. If any information presented was irrelevant, then we believe it was ignored by the raters.[3]

When judgments about sensitivity and accessibility are made, many factors need to be considered. Sensitivity, for example, is not simply a matter of question topic, but is a quality resulting from many variables associated with the question, the survey, and the type of respondents. A minimum of information, as our pilot subjects made clear, is not a solid basis upon which to make a judgment about sensitivity. Raters' confidence in their ability to make a judgment increased with the amount of information at hand.

Subjects responding to survey questions also have a maximum of information. For example, they have knowledge about the exact question wording, the context, the method, and the stated purpose of the survey. Their response to questions occurs within the context of all of this information. Estimates concerning the effect of survey question characteristics on subjects when they respond in surveys are perhaps best made when we possess to the greatest extent possible this same breadth of information.

Returning to the rating process, the raters worked individually, assigning ratings to each question or group of questions from a single study before the next question or study was described. In some cases where a study involved a large number of questions similarly administered, the raters completed their ratings outside of the meeting.[4]

We then did principal-components factor analyses of the sensitivity and accessibility scores of the five raters in order to determine the extent to which the ratings for each dimension indeed reflected a single underlying construct and to assess the degree of similarity among the ratings assigned for each question. We were particularly concerned with the comparability of Wentland's ratings with those of the other judges. The results for accessibility and sensitivity are presented in Table 8.3, with Wentland designated as Rater A.

The means and standard deviations of the accessibility ratings by the five raters are very similar and indicate that, overall, the raters perceived the

---

[3]In retrospect, the presentation of the names of the researchers may have been unnecessary. But most of the raters did not know these authors. Even if they did, this knowledge may have affected their judgments about the overall quality of the research or their estimates of the levels of accuracy obtained. But we did not ask them to provide any of this information.

Since Wentland was familiar with the studies, we were particularly careful to isolate her ratings and to compare them with the ratings provided by others. As reported later in this chapter, there were no important differences. This result supports that information not relevant to judgments of sensitivity and accessibility, for example, information on the levels of accuracy obtained, can be ignored when these judgments are made.

[4]One rater failed to assign an accessibility score to one question. In order to keep that question in the analysis, the missing value was changed to the mean of the accessibility ratings assigned by the other raters to that question.

Table 8.3 Results of the Factor Analyses of the Accessibility and Sensitivity Ratings

Means and Standard Deviations

| | Accessibility | | | Sensibility | |
Rater	Mean	Standard deviation		Mean	Standard deviation
A	4.645	1.079		3.608	1.181
B	4.429	1.382		3.257	1.489
C	4.869	1.052		3.527	1.398
D	4.641	1.171		3.302	1.273
E	4.608	.816		3.176	1.207
N = 245					

Correlation Matrix and Residuals
Accessibility

Rater	A	B	C	D	E
A	.616[a]	.086[b]	.096	.027	.172
B	.553[c]	.664	.087	.105	.071
C	.519	.552	.614	.158	.042
D	.586	.531	.454	.610	.094
E	.447	.571	.575	.521	.621

Sensitivity

Rater	A	B	C	D	E
A	.390[a]	.165[b]	.157	.016	.129
B	.347[c]	.670	.110	.058	.037
C	.326	.523	.598	.090	.051
D	.531	.659	.587	.767	.090
E	.405	.664	.610	.659	.732

Factor Matrix

| Accessibility | | | Sensitivity | |
Rater	Factor 1		Rater	Factor 1
B	.815		D	.876
E	.788		E	.855
A	.785		B	.819
C	.784		C	.773
D	.781		A	.625

Factor Score Coefficient Matrix

| Accessibility | | | Sensitivity | |
Rater	Factor 1		Rater	Factor 1
A	.251		A	.198
B	.261		B	.259
C	.251		C	.245
D	.250		D	.277
E	.252		E	.271

[a]On diagonal, communalities after factor extraction.
[b]Above diagonal, residuals.
[c]Below diagonal, correlation coefficients.

information requested in the questions as being on the accessible end of the rating scale. Further, the correlation matrix reveals that the raters' judgments were highly interrelated.[5]

In the principal-components analysis, 62.5% of the total sample variance could be explained by one factor, which we labeled accessibility. In the factor matrix, the factor loadings for the accessibility factor were large for all five raters. The high communalities (the squares of the factor loadings for this first factor) on the diagonal of the correlation matrix indicate that a large proportion of the variance in each rater's evaluations can be explained by this one factor. To test the goodness of fit of the one-factor model, the correlations among the raters were estimated using just the raters' factor loadings on (correlations with) the first factor.[6] Differences between the estimated and actual correlation coefficients, or residuals, are above the diagonal in the correlation matrix in Table 8.3. They are generally small for a one-factor model: Although 8 of the 10 are greater than .05, only 3 are greater than .10.

Finally, we used regression-method factor score coefficients for each rater (also shown in Table 8.3) to construct a factor score of accessibility for every question. This estimate of the first factor for the accessibility ratings was used in all subsequent analyses to represent the value of accessibility, after partialing out the effects of two variables that could be consistently identified in the studies. These variables and how their effects were statistically partitioned out are described after our discussion of the factor analyses for sensitivity.

The means of the sensitivity ratings for the five raters are also similar and indicate that, on the average, items were viewed as being somewhat sensitive. Raters' sensitivity judgments were also highly correlated. The lowest correlations were those involving Wentland who, unlike the other raters, knew the results of the studies.[7]

The results of the principal-components analysis show that one factor explained 63.1% of the total variance in the ratings of sensitivity, and this first factor had large loadings for all five raters (see Table 8.3). The smallest

---

[5]At the coding stage of the research, Wentland was the only one familiar with the studies. The project had been discussed in a general way with Smith, but he was unfamiliar with any of the particulars or outcomes of the studies, such as the values of the dependent variable.

Because raters' judgments were highly intercorrelated, we concluded that knowledge of the percentage accuracy obtained did not appreciably affect Wentland's judgments. Accuracy rates appear to be less central to these judgments than the many other attributes of the question or survey that were considered. Because it was not a major biasing factor, we elected to retain Wentland's ratings in order to include as much information as possible in our analysis.

[6]The estimated correlation between two raters in a one-factor model is simply the product of their factor loadings on the first factor.

[7]See footnote 5.

loading and communality estimate in the one-factor model is for Wentland. Using the same procedure discussed above with respect to accessibility, the goodness of fit of the one-factor model was tested by comparing the actual correlations among the raters with those estimated with the one-factor model. The residuals, above the diagonal in the correlation matrix for sensitivity in Table 8.3, were again generally small, with 7 of 10 greater than .05, but only 4 of 10 greater than .10. Regression factor-score coefficients were again used to estimate the first factor of sensitivity for each question. Finally sensitivity factor scores were constructed for all questions,[8] and the effects of two identifiable variables were partitioned out before the meta-analyses.

The accessibility of information to respondents in surveys is closely related to the method of administering the questions and the response type, that is, whether a question is binary, calling for a yes or no response, as opposed to, for example, the specification of an amount. The sensitivity of a question likewise is affected by the type of question content and the method of administering the survey. (All of these variables and their coding will be described later in this chapter.) In describing the various study designs and questions to the other raters, Wentland had to include information about these three characteristics of the studies, and this information was no doubt used by the raters in making their evaluations. Unlike many of the other characteristics of the studies, however, information on these three was available for all studies and questions, and we could capture them with fairly objective coding. Furthermore, the three have received a great deal of attention in this report and in the literature, and it seemed advisable to include them separately in the analyses.

We therefore decided to partition out statistically the effects of the survey method and response type on the raters' evaluations of accessibility and the effects of the type of question content and the survey method on sensitivity. The accessibility factor scores were regressed on the method and response-type variables for each question. The unstandardized residuals from this regression, with the effects of method and response type partitioned out, are the estimates of accessibility used in the meta-analyses. Similarly, the net estimates of sensitivity used in the meta-analyses are the residuals from the regression of the sensitivity factor scores on question type and method. As we describe below, the coding of method, response type, and question type varied from analysis to analysis because of small or empty cells in the design. Consequently, the residuals were calculated separately for each analysis.

---

[8]Internal-consistency estimates of the reliability of the accessibility and sensitivity factor scores were .8802 and .89221, respectively, using Heise and Bohrnstedt's index for weighted scales (as cited in Smith, 1974); and .8562 and .85749 using Cronbach's index for an unequally weighted scale (Formula 29 in Smith, 1974).

Study Date

That the year in which a study was conducted may have affected the degree of response accuracy was suggested by Light & Pillemer (1984). Since a great deal of attention has been given to survey research methodology over the years and many suggestions to reduce response error have been made, the percentages of accurate responses to questions of all types may have increased over time. The year of each study was included as an independent variable to explore this possibility.

The year in which the research was actually conducted was the first choice to represent this variable. In 100 cases, this date was used. When the research date was not available, other dates used were the publication date, used in 47 cases; the date the research article was received for publication, used for 4 questions; or the date the research paper was presented at a conference, used in 94 instances. In a choice situation, the date selected was the one that appeared to be closest to the time when the data were collected.[9]

Response Type

Many survey questions in the studies we analyzed called for a yes or no response, while others required the specification of an amount. In certain cases involving questions about amounts, categories were provided for respondents. In other cases, respondents provided the information in open-ended responses. Standards for determining the accuracy of amounts varied greatly, from the exact amount to accuracy within specified ranges. While the supposed effect of these different standards was probably reflected in the accessibility ratings, we could only code as a separate variable whether a question was framed to elicit a yes or no response or a quantity. Binary and not binary questions were coded 0 and 1, respectively, so that the estimated effects of this variable in the analyses indicate how nonbinary questions increase or decrease response accuracy relative to the accuracy of binary questions.

Method

Survey method is frequently cited in the literature as an important influence on response accuracy. In many instances, comparisons are made between accuracy rates obtained using different methods. Those methods that ensure respondents' anonymity or the confidentiality of replies are believed to produce more truthful replies, especially to sensitive behavior questions. Much

---

[9]Four questions included in this analysis were from a study by Robins (1966) that was conducted over a 6-year period, from 1955 to 1960. Since it appeared that the bulk of the interviews were conducted in the early stages of the project (p. 37), the date selected for this study was 1957.

attention has been given to the development of methods of this type, for example, the random response method. On the other hand, the probing of skillful interviewers in face-to-face situations may assist the recall of information or events. Accessibility may also be increased when questionnaires are left with respondents, allowing for consultation with others or with records.

Four methods were used to ask the questions included in this analysis: face-to-face interview, questionnaire, telephone interview, and random response. These four methods were coded in a categorical variable that was represented by dummy variables in some of the analyses.[10]

Differences within methods were also found in the various studies. These differences include group versus individual administration of a questionnaire, structured versus unstructured interview, and paid versus unpaid respondents. Altogether, differences within a method were used in 5 studies involving 25 questions. Although not reflected in the gross method ratings, these differences are assumed to be included in the sensitivity and accessibility ratings.

Socially Desirable Response Direction

Parry & Crossley (1950) suggested that high levels of accuracy will be obtained from questions "where invalidity is basically in the direction of exaggeration" (p. 75), and which involve behaviors performed by a large number of the respondents. The authors noted that the low level of invalidity in those cases is artifactual, occurring simply because there is a smaller group of persons likely to give incorrect replies. Cahalan (1968) followed up on this reasoning and found a fairly high positive rank-order correlation ($r = .65$) between the percentages of persons who performed the behavior and the percentages of accurate responses for 13 survey questions analyzed in his report, all of which involved what we characterized as a positive socially desirable response. We excluded one of those 13 questions, because it was actually a combination of 2 questions, and found a significant positive Pearson correlation ($r = .69$, $df = 10$, $p < .01$) between response accuracy and performance for the remaining 12 items.[11]

---

[10]Although method was clearly specified and therefore easily coded for most questions, in three studies, a combination of methods was used. Sobell *et al.* (1974) used a questionnaire and then a face-to-face interview on the same questions. In the two studies by Ferber *et al.* (1969a,b), certain respondents were personally interviewed, while others were given a questionnaire in addition to an interview. The eight questions from these three studies were included in the face-to-face method category.

[11]The percentages used by Cahalan (1968) in his calculation were somewhat different from the percentages that we used because we excluded the "don't remember" or "no answer" responses, thereby reducing the size of the respondent group.

For questions to which a "no" response is socially desirable, it follows that high incidence of performance among the respondents will most likely be associated with low levels of response accuracy, because performers will be motivated to deny the behavior. On the other hand, low performance incidence will produce high rates of accuracy because the socially desirable answers would be truthful denials.

Support for this hypothesis was found in an exploration involving the 28 deviant behavior items and 5 sexual behavior items included in Clark & Tifft's (1966) report. Respondents were to report the frequency with which they had engaged in the various socially undesirable behaviors. Pearson correlations between the percentages of persons who had actually performed the behavior and the percentages who provided truthful responses were significant and negative for both the deviant behavior items ($r = -.874, df = 26, p < .001$) and the sexual behavior questions ($r = -.891, df = 3, p < .05$).

We decided to include a scoring of social desirability so that we could explore both the independent effect on accuracy of the direction of socially desirable responding and its possible interaction with the incidence of behavior performance.

Questions were coded into one of three categories, represented in some analyses by dummy variables. Those questions for which it was socially desirable to respond "no," or to minimize in the case of nonbinary questions, were assigned to the "undesirable" category. An example of these questions is Weiss's (1968) question concerning whether the respondent's child had ever had to repeat a grade in school. Questions for which the socially desirable response was to say "yes," or to exaggerate, were coded as "desirable," for example, voting behavior questions.

When it was not possible to make a determination as to the socially desirable response direction, the question was coded as "mixed" or "indeterminate." Examples of this category include age questions, depending on the age mix of the respondents. While older respondents may claim to be younger, young respondents may overstate their age. This third category was also used to identify questions for which the direction of social desirability was either not clear or not a relevant issue. Hyman's (1944) questions to storekeepers concerning the receipt of government posters exemplify this type of question. Another example is a question in Ito's (1963) report concerning the amount of monthly car payments. Although it might be socially desirable to overstate this amount, thereby increasing the car's value, it may also be socially desirable to understate so as to communicate less indebtedness. Therefore, we decided to assign this question to the indeterminate category.[12]

---

[12]Although coding on this variable required making a judgment, this process was relatively unproblematic. However, in certain cases, colleagues were consulted and judgments pooled.

To check our judgments of the direction of the socially desirable response, we compared assigned codes with the percentages of overstatements and understatements for the respective questions. For questions where the socially desirable response is either to say "yes" or to exaggerate, error should mainly take the form of overstatements. Where the socially desirable response is either to say "no" or to minimize, invalid answers should mainly be underreports. Because of the many possible reasons for assigning the indeterminate code, we were not able to make predictions concerning the distribution of error for those questions.

Because error can be in only one direction for reverse record check sample questions, this check was performed on just the general sample questions. Three questions were excluded because there were no performers and error was possible in only one direction. Of the 41 general sample questions for which the judgment had been made that it was socially desirable to say "yes" or exaggerate, 36 or about 88% of the questions had more overreports than underreports. In another two instances, the number of overreports and underreports was identical. Of the 112 questions where a "no" or minimizing response was judged to be socially desirable, 40 or almost 36% of the questions had more underreports than overreports. Another 36, or about 32% of the questions, had equal numbers of overstatements and understatements. For the remaining 36 questions, our judgment of negative socially desirable response direction coding was not supported by the distribution of overreports and underreports. Twenty-eight of these questions, however, were from the study by Sobell & Sobell (1978), in which the numbers of respondents were very small (N's = 11, 12, 13, or 14) and the percentages of accurate and inaccurate respondents consequently are very unstable.

We concluded that these results supported our socially desirable response direction coding for those questions coded as desirable. The results are mixed for questions we coded as undesirable. It seems clear from the content of the questions, however, that the behaviors are socially undesirable. False claims or exaggerations of negative behavior, then, are not unusual in these data and may occur more frequently in surveys than commonly believed.[13]

Prevalence

As we have noted, the socially desirable direction of a response to a question and the incidence of performance of the related behavior among the respondents, or prevalence, may interact to affect response accuracy. We included

---

[13]These type responses are also discussed by Hessing *et al.* (1988).

prevalence as an independent variable to investigate this interactive effect and its possible main effect. Prevalence was represented by the percentages of respondents to particular questions who were involved in the behavior or subject under investigation. In cases where all of the respondents were involved, as in the 86 reverse record check questions, prevalence was 100%. In 89 of the 159 other cases, information concerning prevalence was not available.[14]

Question Type

To facilitate the qualitative review of the questions included in this report, questions were grouped into 10 subject areas, presumably differing in levels of threat or sensitivity. Ordered from least to most sensitive, these were descriptive information, various events and behaviors, attendance and absenteeism, hospitalization episodes, cigarette smoking, voting behavior, alcohol-related behavior, deviant behavior, sexual behavior, and financial matters. Through a sequence of analyses, we ultimately reduced these to three categories of question type that were used in the meta-analyses.

Three issues concerning question type were explored. These were (1) whether question type had a significant effect on question accuracy, independent of the effects of other variables, such as question sensitivity; (2) whether each question type category was distinct in terms of its association with accuracy; and (3) whether any further collapsing of question type categories was appropriate for pragmatic reasons. The last question was a corollary to the second question and arose because of a concern about the small number of cases in certain categories. Another reason for investigating the possibility of collapsing categories was that a reduced number of question type categories would result in a decreased number of empty cells in a factor/factor interaction matrix.

Intuitively, it seemed that certain categories were similar in their levels of sensitivity and that perhaps three new groups of questions could be formed, focused around the descriptive, deviant, and financial categories. Statistical support for this regrouping came from two analyses of covariance, performed with percentage accuracy of responses to each question as the dependent variable and sensitivity, accessibility, study date, response type, method, so-

---

[14]Prevalence rates are not based upon the self-reported data. Rather, they are independent estimates based upon external criteria. In many of the studies reviewed, prevalence information was not available because percentage accuracy figures were not broken down into performers and nonperformers.

cially desirable response direction, sample type (general or reverse record check), and question type as the independent variables.[15]

With eight categories in the analysis, the main effect for question type was not significant.[16] From an examination of the adjusted deviations from the grand mean for the eight categories in the multiple-classification part of the analysis of covariance, it appeared that they could be combined into two groups (see Table 8.4, Analysis A).[17] The first group, labeled Descriptive Information and Behavior, consisted of descriptive information, attendance and absenteeism, and voting behavior questions, which had higher mean percentages of accuracy than the grand or overall mean. In contrast, lower-than-average means were found for questions concerning hospitalization episodes, alcohol-related behavior, deviant behavior, sexual behavior, and financial matters. Except for financial matters, all of those question type categories were combined to form a second group, labeled Deviant and Personal Behavior. We decided to retain the Financial Matters category as a third major group because financial questions tended to ask for detailed amounts and seemed to be of a somewhat different character than the other questions included in the Deviant and Personal Behavior category.

To confirm the reasonableness of these combinations, we did an analysis of covariance with the three new categories of the question type variable. The main effect for question type was once again significant ($F = 3.793$, $df = 2$, $p < .05$), while the results of the multiple classification analysis were consistent with the prior findings (see Table 8.4, Analysis B). The Descriptive Information and Behavior category had a small positive adjusted deviation from the grand mean, while the other two categories had similar slightly negative adjusted deviations.

---

[15]As previously noted, the sensitivity scores used in the various analyses described in this chapter were the residual scores resulting from the regression of the sensitivity factor scores on method and question type. The number of categories in the question type variable used in these regressions corresponded to the number of categories in the question type variable being used in the target analyses.

Prevalence was not included in this analysis because of the large number of missing values.

[16]Because of their small numbers, the two questions in the Cigarette Smoking category and the five questions from the Various Events and Behaviors category were distributed into other appropriate question type categories. We decided that the cigarette smoking questions and the questions about childrens' school failures could be classified as deviant behavior items, while the questions on the receipt and display of store posters could be considered within the Descriptive Information category.

[17]The adjusted deviations in Table 8.4 are from the weighted analyses. For a description of the weighting procedure and its rationale, see the concluding section of this chapter.

Table 8.4 Multiple Classification Analyses Results for Question Type and Sample Type Variables

Variable	Sample size		Deviations adjusted for factors and covariates
	Unweighted	Weighted	
Analysis A			
Question Type: 8 Categories			
1. Descriptive information	16	37	3.64
2. Attendance and absenteeism	5	6	8.57
3. Hospitalization episodes	12	23	−.22
4. Voting behavior	24	81	1.79
5. Alcohol-related behavior	80	6	−1.29
6. Deviant behavior	41	16	−.97
7. Sexual behavior	8	1	−6.78
8. Financial matters	58	74	−3.91
Total	244	244	
Sample Type			
0. Reverse record check	85	100	−5.29
1. General	159	144	3.66
Total	244	244	
Analysis B			
Question Type: 3 Categories			
1. Descriptive information and			3.63
behavior	45	124	−3.91
2. Deviant and personal behavior	141	46	−3.60
3. Financial matters	58	74	
Total	244	244	
Sample Type			
0. Reverse record check	85	100	−4.98
1. General	159	144	3.44
Total	244	244	

Formation of Question Subsets

Questions were broadly categorized as involving either a reverse record check or a general sample design. As previously noted, a reverse record check design in this report is one in which 100% of the respondents were involved in the behavior or subject under investigation, while all other cases were considered general sample ones.[18]

---

[18]For a further explanation of reverse record check samples, see footnote 1 in Chapter 2. In these meta-analyses, the two tax questions from the report by Hessing _et al._ (1988), in which respondents were preselected nonevaders, were coded as general sample questions, with 0% prevalence. Only questions assigned 100% prevalence were considered reverse record check sample ones.

We have already discussed that the percentages of accuracy for reverse record check samples are not directly comparable to the percentages for general samples because of the inherent understatement or overstatement of error in the former. Accordingly, we decided to perform separate analyses on the questions from each of these design types. Support for this decision was found in the multiple classification analysis results from the analyses of variance carried out and described in the discussion of the question type variable (see Table 8.4). There was a significant main effect for the dichotomous variable sample type in both Analyses A and B ($F = 8.915$, $df = 1$, $p < .01$, and $F = 9.072$, $df = 1$, $p < .01$, respectively). Reverse record check sample questions were consistently associated with lower-than-average accuracy, while percentages of accuracy for general sample questions were somewhat higher than average.

Of the 159 questions which used general samples, prevalence information was available for only 70 questions. In order to assess as many general sample questions as possible, the prevalence variable was omitted from the first regression analysis. A second analysis of the general sample items with prevalence among the independent variables included just those questions with prevalence values.

Variable Selection for the Analyses

Analysis I: All General Sample Questions

With respect to the four categorical independent variables — response type, method, socially desirable response direction, and question type — the one-way and two-way joint frequency distributions of these variables were examined to ascertain whether there were sufficient numbers of questions, first, to permit the retention of all categories of these variables in the analysis and, second, to support any analysis of two-way interaction effects. The examination of the frequency distributions of the 159 general sample questions revealed small numbers of cases in three categories: the telephone ($N = 2$) and random response ($N = 1$) categories for the method variable and the indeterminate ($N = 4$) category for socially desirable response direction.[19] Further, in the two-way cross-tabulations of these categorical variables with all levels included, each distribution had at least two empty cells.[20]

---

[19]Unless otherwise noted, all procedures were weighted as explained at the end of this chapter.

[20]The questions included in this report represent the pattern of research in the area of survey response validity under investigation. Unfortunately, this pattern did not produce anything approaching a balanced design. In all three of the meta-analyses, the presence of categories with small numbers of cases and empty cells is an indication that researchers have tended to focus on certain survey question attributes and to give little attention to others.

The three categories with small numbers of cases were eliminated, resulting in a total of 149 general sample questions available for analysis. Method and socially desirable response direction became two-category dummy variables (see Table 8.5). The reference categories for response type, method, and social desirability were binary, face to face, and negative, respectively. The only nondichotomous variable was question type, which consisted of three categories. Two dummy variables were created to represent this variable with financial matters as the reference category.

In the joint frequency distributions of this new group of questions by the categorical variables, there were two instances in which sufficient numbers of cases were included in the cells to allow for an assessment of interactions

Table 8.5 Frequencies of Questions by Categories of the Four Categorical Independent Variables, by Question Groups

Variable and category	All general sample questions[a] (N = 149)		General sample questions with prevalence information[a] (N = 68)		Reverse record check sample questions[b] (N = 78)	
	Unweighted	Weighted	Unweighted	Weighted	Unweighted	Weighted
Response type						
Binary	51	137	34	65	38	27
Not binary	98	12	34	3	40	51
Method						
Face to face	31	122	25	59	63	67
Questionnaire	118	27	43	9	15	11
Socially desirable response direction						
Negative	115	31	43	11	33	13
Positive	34	118	25	57	28	36
Indeterminate	—	—	—	—	17	29
Question type						
Descriptive information and behavior	28	113	22	55	8	11
Deviant and personal behavior	115	25	40	8	21	15
Financial matters	6	11	6	5	49	51[c]

[a]Without questions that fell into the Indeterminate Socially Desirable Response Direction category and the Telephone and Random Response Method categories. See text for explanation.

[b]Without questions that fell into the Telephone and Random Response Method categories. See text for explanation.

[c]The individual Ns do not add up to the total N because of rounding errors.

between the variables.[21] These instances were method by socially desirable response direction and method by question type. Three new variables representing these interactions were created for inclusion in the regression analysis.

Descriptive statistics for the four continuous variables, including the dependent variable, are presented in Table 8.6.[22] Ten additional variables were also created representing the interactions between the categorical variables and sensitivity and accessibility. Overall, a total of 21 independent variables were now available for analysis.

Analysis II: General Sample Questions with Prevalence Information

Seventy of the general sample questions were selected for a separate analysis because of the availability of prevalence information for that group. Prevalence refers to the percentages of respondents who had performed the behavior or who possessed the item in question.

Because this group of questions is a subset of the group of questions used in the first analysis, similar findings were expected and obtained concerning which categories of the discrete variables could be included in the meta-analysis. Within the unweighted frequency distributions of these 70 questions by the four categorical variables, there was one instance of an empty category, the random response category for method. Further, there was only 1 question in each of two categories: the telephone category for the method variable and the indeterminate socially desirable response direction category. In the weighted frequency distributions, those two categories virtually disappeared. Therefore, we decided to eliminate them, as well as the random response method category, from the analysis. The frequency distributions for the categorical variables for the resulting group of 68 questions are presented in Table 8.5. In this analysis, as in Analysis I, method and socially desirable response direction both were reduced to two-category variables. Question type remained a three-category variable, represented by two dummy variables.

The two-way cross-tabulations of the 68 questions, according to the categorical variables, revealed that in no instance was there a sufficient number of cases in all cells to support an analysis of interaction effects. In four of the

---

[21]The cross-tabulations mentioned in this section and matrices of correlations are available upon request from the principal author.

[22]As previously explained, the sensitivity and accessibility variables used in these regression analyses were the unstandardized residuals from the regressions of the sensitivity factor scores on method and question type, and the accessibility factor scores on method and response type. These residuals were calculated separately for each question subset. The number of levels of the categorical variables used to create these residuals corresponded to the number of levels used in the respective analyses.

Table 8.6 Descriptive Statistics for the Dependent Variable and the Continuous Independent Variables, by Question Group

Question group	N	Variable	Mean[a]	Standard deviation[a]	Minimum	Maximum
All general sample questions	149[b]	Percentage accurate	83.79 (81.52)	10.84 (17.15)	23.10	100.00
		Sensitivity	.02 (−.00)	.63 (.77)	−2.48	1.87
		Accessibility	.00 (−.00)	.96 (.84)	−2.43	1.73
		Study date	1963.18 (1970.02)	12.67 (8.92)	1944	1984
General sample questions with prevalence information	68[b]	Percentage accurate	83.90 (81.29)	10.31 (14.73)	32.50	100.00
		Sensitivity	.04 (.00)	.61 (.86)	−2.23	2.13
		Accessibility	.02 (−.00)	.99 (1.03)	−2.43	1.55
		Study date	1962.56 (1963.60)	12.92 (9.59)	1944	1984
		Prevalence	50.10 (39.33)	21.07 (27.64)	0.00	96.20
Reverse record check sample questions	78[c]	Percentage accurate	61.40 (65.73)	24.01 (19.61)	10.40	98.10
		Sensitivity	−.27 (−.00)	.79 (.87)	−2.15	1.64
		Accessibility	−.22 (.00)	1.12 (.91)	−3.25	1.90
		Study date	1957.25 (1959.96)	6.05 (7.78)	1944	1984

[a]Unweighted statistic in parentheses.
[b]See footnote [a] in Table 8.5.
[c]See footnote [b] in Table 8.5.

joint frequency distributions, there was at least one empty cell, while at least one cell in each of the two other distributions had only two questions.[23]

---

[23]The two joint frequency distributions which had two questions in at least one of the cells were method by socially desirable response direction and method by question type.

Descriptive statistics for the four continuous independent variables and the dependent variable are presented in Table 8.6. Fifteen additional variables were also created to represent the interactions between the four categorical variables and three continuous variables — sensitivity, accessibility, and prevalence — resulting in a total of 24 independent variables to be included in the meta-analysis.

Analysis III: Reverse Record Check Sample Questions

In the unweighted frequency distributions of the 85 reverse record check sample questions by the four categorical variables, the telephone and random response categories for method again contained only a small number of cases, 5 and 2 respectively. These numbers were reduced to 4 and 0 in the weighted distributions (rounded to the nearest whole number). Therefore, we decided to eliminate those two categories from further analyses. The frequency distributions for the remaining 78 questions are presented in Table 8.5. Since socially desirable response direction had three categories, two dummy variables were created to represent that variable, with indeterminate questions as the reference category.

Two of the two-way distributions of the categorical variables had sufficient numbers of questions in all of the cells to test interaction effects between the variables. These were response type by socially desirable response direction and method by socially desirable response direction. Four dummy variables representing these interactions were created by multiplying together the dummy variables for the corresponding categorical ones.

Descriptive statistics for the dependent variable and the three continuous independent variables are displayed in Table 8.6. The inclusion in the regression analysis of the interactions between the categorical variables and both sensitivity and accessibility required the creation of 12 additional variables. Altogether, a total of 25 independent variables was available for analysis.

Weighted Regression Analyses of Percentage Accuracy

In the analyses for reducing the number of question types and in the meta-analyses themselves, we used weighted data to account for the number of respondents in each of the studies or questions in our analyses. There was extreme variation in the numbers of respondents answering the questions. Questions with few respondents were a source of concern because percentages of accuracy for these questions are relatively unstable. Another reason for concern was the large number of questions that had these small numbers of respondents. For example, just over 29%, or 72 of the 245 questions selected for this analysis came from a single study, that of Sobell & Sobell (1978), where the numbers of respondents were quite small, ranging from 11 to 14. We therefore weighted the data to insure that the contribution of each question would be in proportion to the number of subjects involved in any analysis where the dependent variable was percentage of accurate responses. The weighting formula was simply

$$W_i = (N_i / \Sigma\, N_j)\, K, \quad j = 1 \ldots K,$$

where W_i is the weight for question i, N_i is the number of respondents asked question i, N_j is the number asked question j, and K is the number of questions in a given analysis. This weighting assures that the weighted number of questions is the same as the actual number of questions. We should stress that the weights were calculated separately for each analysis we report.

In most studies, the exact number of persons answering the questions was provided or could be calculated based on the data presented. However, in Cannell & Fowler's (1963) study of hospitalization episodes, the number of respondents was not given for 10 of the 12 questions examined. These 10 questions, 5 in each of two survey methods, concerned the particular details of a hospitalization. We assumed that these questions were addressed only to those persons who admitted having been hospitalized, and we assumed that the percentages of respondents truthfully acknowledging hospitalizations were roughly equivalent to the number of episodes correctly reported (there was a slightly higher number of episodes than people for both methods). These percentages of respondents were therefore used to obtain the number of respondents for these 10 questions.

As we have already noted in our discussion of the dummy variables, we generally used ordinary least-squares regression for the meta-analyses. Through dummy variables for main effects and interactions, this analysis parallels an analysis of covariance, except that it more readily allows for interactions between categorical and continuous variables. Also, it provides estimates of coefficients that are substantively interpretable rather than just tests of their significance.

9

Meta-Analysis: Results and Discussion

Analysis I: All General Sample Questions

Results

This first analysis includes all of the general sample questions, that is, those that were not reverse record check. Prevalence could not be included as it was missing for many of the questions (see footnote 14 in Chapter 8).

Results of the regression analysis are presented in Table 9.1. The analysis was conducted in two stages. Following the traditional approach for analysis of variance studies, the eight main variables were entered together in the first stage. All were significant, and together they accounted for approximately 63% of the variance in percentage accuracy of responses.

In the next stage, the 13 interaction variables were subjected to a stepwise selection procedure to see if any of them had an effect over and above the main effects. Two interactions entered the equations: nonbinary response type by sensitivity and questionnaire method by deviant/personal question type. With the questionnaire by deviant/personal interaction in the equation, the main effect of the questionnaire method dropped to insignificance. Following the hierarchical principle of retaining main effects associated with interaction variables, however, we kept it in the final model. With the addition of the two significant interaction variables, the model explained 66% of the variation in percentage of accurate responses (adjusted R^2).[1]

---

[1] Two questions were identified as influential using Cook's distance measure. These were Sobell & Sobell's (1978) question addressed to 12 court-referred outpatient alcoholics concerning the number of drunk driving convictions, and Clark & Tifft's (1966) question (*continues*)

Table 9.1 Variables in the Equation for Percentage of Accurate Response: Analysis I: General Sample Questions without Prevalence

	Coefficients		
Independent variable	Unstandardized	Standardized	t test
Question type: Deviant/Personal	−14.05	−.49	−3.71***
Question type: Descriptive	12.84	.51	5.60***
Accessibility	7.87	.70	13.24***
Sensitivity	−5.37	−.31	−4.60***
Nonbinary response	−8.26	−.21	−2.86**
Positive social desirability	−16.95	−.64	−5.84***
Study date	.14	.16	2.76**
Nonbinary by sensitivity	8.86	.21	3.85***
Questionnaire method by deviant/personal	10.69	.33	2.59*
Method	.98	.03	.39
Constant	−187.12		−1.87
R^2, .681			
Adjusted R^2, .657			
Standard error, 6.343			
F (10, 138), 29.409***			

Notes: $* p < .05$; $** p < .01$; $*** p < .001$

Discussion

An examination of the standardized regression coefficients revealed that the most potent variable in the regression equation was accessibility, which was positively related to response accuracy. The second most influential variable was positive social desirability, which had a negative association with accuracy. That is, those questions to which a "yes" response was socially desirable tended to be less accurate than those questions to which the socially desirable response was "no."

The dummy variables for question type, both significant, had equal standing in the regression equation, but with opposite signs. As expected, the descriptive information and behavior questions tended to be more accurate

---

(*continued*) addressed to 40 male college undergraduate students concerning the frequency with which, since entering high school, they had skipped school without a legitimate excuse. However, the results of the regression analysis without those two questions were virtually identical to the results for the entire set of questions. The failure of the two questions to affect the analysis is attributable to the small number of respondents in each case, which would reduce the influence of the questions in a weighted analysis. For this entire group of questions, the average number of respondents was approximately 197.

than questions in the deviant and personal behavior and financial matters categories. As compared to the other categories, deviant and personal behavior questions were less accurate.

For one of the two dummy variables for question type, deviant/personal, there was also a significant interaction with the questionnaire method. Although the questionnaire method by itself had no significant effect on accuracy, the positive association between response accuracy and this interaction variable suggests that, for deviant questions, the survey method did make a difference. That is, even though deviant and personal behavior questions were less accurate overall than questions in the descriptive information and behavior and financial matters categories, more accurate responses to questions on deviant and personal behavior were obtained with questionnaires than in face-to-face interviews.

Perhaps no survey question characteristic has received as much attention in the literature as question sensitivity, which is widely believed to be the most important variable affecting response accuracy. However, in this analysis, question sensitivity, although significant, was not the dominant variable. The negative association between sensitivity and response accuracy was as expected.

There was also a significant main effect for nonbinary response type and a significant interaction between nonbinary responses and sensitivity. Overall, binary questions tended to be more accurate than nonbinary questions. However, the interaction suggests that for particularly sensitive questions, greater response accuracy was obtained when questions were posed in a nonbinary format.

The relationship between study date and percentage of accurate responses was positive, indicating that more recent studies tended to have higher accuracy rates. This finding may reflect improvements over time in survey design or methodology.

Analysis II: General Sample Questions with Prevalence Information

Results

The first analysis did not include the prevalence characteristic because it was not available for many of the questions. This second analysis is limited to the subset of general questions with prevalence data. The variables considered are the same as in Analysis I, with prevalence added.

The regression analysis results are presented in Table 9.2. Proceeding in two stages as in Analysis I, the main variables were first entered together. In all, these nine variables accounted for about 73% of the variation in percentage accuracy of responses. Six variables were significant: accessibility, positive social desirability, sensitivity, both descriptive and deviant/personal question types, and study date.

In the next stage, the 15 interaction variables were made available for inclusion through a stepwise selection procedure. Only the interaction between deviant/personal questions and prevalence entered the regression equation, increasing the percentage of variation explained to approximately 84%. With the inclusion of this interaction variable, prevalence, which previously had virtually no effect, was now significant. A dramatic change also occurred with respect to the unstandardized regression coefficient for the main effect of deviant/personal questions. At the end of the first stage of the analysis, this coefficient was -9.162, while at the end of the second stage, its coefficient was 17.307.[2]

Discussion

Eight variables remained in the regression equation. These included all four continuous variables, the dummy variables for the two categories of question type, positive social desirability, and the variable representing the interaction between prevalence and deviant/personal questions. Together they accounted for 81% of the variance in percentage of accurate response (adjusted R^2).

The introduction of prevalence to the analysis of general sample questions had an important effect. According to the standardized regression coefficients, or beta weights, the interaction variable was the most powerful vari-

---

[2]Using Cook's distance measure, 4 questions were identified as influential. All 4 questions were from Clark & Tifft's (1966) study in which 40 male college undergraduate students were asked about the frequency with which they had performed various deviant and sexual behaviors since entering high school. The influential questions were how often a respondent had driven a motor vehicle at extreme speeds, skipped school without a legitimate excuse, taken little things that didn't belong to him, and had sex relations with a person of the opposite sex who was not his wife. A regression analysis performed without these 4 questions produced results almost identical to the results for all 68 questions. One explanation involves the relatively small number of respondents for each of these 4 questions compared to 397, which was the approximate average number of respondents for the entire subset of 68 questions. In a weighted analysis, the contribution of the four influential questions was minimized.

The variable representing the interaction between socially desirable response direction and sensitivity failed to enter the regression equation, but was close to being significant ($t = -1.869$, $p = .0666$) and clearly would have been included in the model had there been an additional step. To assess the effect of the inclusion of that interaction variable in the model, we performed a separate regression analysis where socially desirable response direction by sensitivity was entered together with the 8 significant variables. The result was that the interaction variable essentially replaced sensitivity in the equation. For reasons of generality and parsimony, we elected to retain sensitivity instead.

Table 9.2 Variables in the Equation for Percentage of Accurate Response: Analysis II: General Sample Questions with Prevalence

Independent variable	Coefficients		
	Unstandardized	Standardized	t test
Question type: Deviant/personal	17.79	.56	3.27**
Question type: Descriptive	12.95	.50	5.67***
Accessibility	5.74	.55	7.30***
Sensitivity	−5.71	−.34	−4.84***
Prevalence	.16	.33	3.6***
Positive social desirability	−14.05	−.51	−4.73***
Study date	.11	.13	2.01*
Deviant/personal by prevalence	−.61	−.81	−6.28***
Constant	−129.42		−1.26
R^2, .834			
Adjusted R^2, .811			
Standard error, 4.483			
F (8, 59), 36.925***			

Notes: * $p < .05$; ** $p < .01$; *** $p < .001$

able and was negatively associated with response accuracy. The two dummy variables for question type were also strong. In contrast to the results in the first analysis with all of the general sample questions, both of the dummy variables for question type had a positive association with accuracy. The above findings, however, must be understood in the context of prevalence and the interaction of prevalence with deviant/personal types of questions.

Before the interaction variable entered the regression equation, the unstandardized regression coefficients for the dummy variables for question type followed the pattern found in Analysis I. That is, the coefficient for the variable comparing descriptive information and behavior questions with the other two categories was positive, while the coefficient for the variable comparing the deviant and personal behavior questions with all others was negative. By itself, prevalence was not significant. While the inclusion of the interaction variable did not markedly affect the values for descriptive types of questions, the unstandardized regression coefficient for deviant/personal questions became strongly positive. Prevalence became significant, with a positive effect on accuracy. However, when prevalence, the dummy variables for question type, and the interaction variable are considered together in the regression equation, descriptive information and behavior questions continue to be the most accurate overall, followed by financial matters questions. For those question types, prevalence and accuracy were positively related. For the least accurate deviant and personal questions, the effect of prevalence on response accuracy was reversed. Questions about low prevalence behavior tended to be more accurate than questions about high prevalence behavior. That is, questions about deviant and personal behavior were responded to more accurately the fewer the number of respondents who had actually engaged in the behavior.

The finding that prevalence and response accuracy are inversely related for deviant and personal behavior questions and positively associated for descriptive information and behavior and financial matters questions recalls the explorations by Parry & Crossley (1950) and Cahalan (1968) concerning the effect of behavior prevalence on accuracy. To summarize, the researchers proposed that for questions to which invalid responses tend to be exaggerations, accuracy and prevalence will be positively correlated. In other words, the greater the number of respondents who had actually performed the desirable behavior, the fewer would be able to provide an untruthful "yes" response. In fact, as previously discussed, we found a significant positive Pearson correlation ($r = .69$, $df = 10$, $p < .01$) between prevalence and accuracy for 12 socially desirable behavior items included in the survey analyzed in Cahalan's report.[3]

Extending this reasoning to questions for which the socially desirable response was "no," we hypothesized that as the number of respondents who had engaged in the behavior decreases, accuracy increases, simply because there are fewer persons motivated to supply an untruthful "no" response. In support of this hypothesis, we found a significant negative Pearson correlation between prevalence and accuracy for both the 28 deviant behavior items ($r = -.874$, $df = 26$, $p < .001$), and the 5 sexual behavior items ($r = -.891$, $df = 3$, $p < .05$) included in Clark & Tifft's (1966) study.

However, according to the results of this meta-analysis, question type rather than socially desirable response direction emerged as the variable that mediated the relationship between response accuracy and prevalence. Further support for this conclusion was found when Pearson correlation coefficients were computed between prevalence and percentage of accurate responses, first within the categories defined by the socially desirable response direction and then within the categories defined by the type of question. Unfortunately, the two dimensions have been confounded in many studies, and there are few questions that can be used to distinguish between the two sets of correlations. However, the correlations between prevalence and accuracy tend to be larger within the categories of question type than within the categories defined by the direction of social desirability. Certainly this is one area in

---

[3]See the discussion of these items and also of Clark & Tifft's (1966) study in Chapters 3 and 4. Further, see the discussion in Chapter 8 of the independent variable, socially desirable response direction.

which further research is needed with comparisons designed specifically to disentangle these two dimensions.

As expected, the remaining variables—accessibility, socially desirable response direction, sensitivity, and study date—followed much the same pattern found in the first analysis with respect to both the direction and the relative strength of their effects on response accuracy. The effects of both accessibility and study date were positive, while those for sensitivity and positive social desirability were negative.

Analysis III: Reverse Record Check Sample Questions

Results

The third analysis is of the data for those questions classified as reverse record check, that is, those questions for which all subjects had performed the behavior or had the characteristic.

The regression analysis results for this set of questions are presented in Table 9.3. As with the other question subsets, the analysis was conducted in two stages. First, the 3 continuous variables and the 6 variables representing the categorical variables were entered together. Almost 56% of the variation in percent accurate responses was accounted for by those variables. However, of the variables in the equation, only accessibility and non-binary response type were significant.

In the second stage, the 16 interaction variables were made available for inclusion in the regression equation through a stepwise selection process. Five interaction terms entered during this stage. By order of entry, these were nonbinary response by positive social desirability,[4] nonbinary response by accessibility, positive social desirability by accessibility, negative social desirability by accessibility, and questionnaire method by positive social desirability. With these five interactions also in the equation, three additional main effects were significant: deviant/personal question type, positive social desirability, and study date. Thus, the final equation contained 10 significant variables, which together explained about 69% of the variation in response accuracy (adjusted R^2).

Discussion

Of the 10 variables in the equation at the last step of the regression analysis, 5 were interaction variables. Three variables were prominent in the equation:

---

[4]Recall that in the reverse record check sample there were enough questions to include the indeterminate social desirability category. This was the reference category, so that effects of both the positive and the negative social desirability dummy variables are relative to that for the indeterminate category.

Table 9.3 Variables in the Equation for Percentage of Accurate Response: Analysis III: Reverse Record Check Sample Questions

Independent variable	Coefficients		
	Unstandardized	Standardized	t test
Question type: Deviant/personal	16.26	.27	2.94**
Accessibility	32.64	1.53	6.08***
Nonbinary response	−11.04	−.22	−1.89*
Positive social desirability	21.52	.45	3.30**
Study date	−1.30	−.33	−3.65***
Nonbinary by accessibility	−18.78	−.83	−3.83***
Nonbinary by positive social desirability	−44.60	−.82	−5.03***
Positive social desirability by accessibility	−15.71	−.55	−3.79***
Negative social desirability by accessibility	−15.88	−.26	−2.97**
Questionnaire by positive social desirability	34.46	.27	3.58***
Constant	−2617.39		3.76***
R^2, .726			
Adjusted R^2, .685			
Standard error, 13.466			
F (10, 67), 17.771***			

Notes: $* p < .05$; $** p < .01$; $*** p < .001$

7 of the 10 significant variables were either their main effects or interactions which involved them. The three key variables were accessibility, response type, and socially desirable response direction, particularly the dummy variable comparing positive social responses with indeterminate ones. For these reverse record check sample questions, the sensitivity of a question had no effect on response accuracy.

Using the standardized regression coefficients as indicators of the relative importance of the variables in the model, accessibility was clearly dominant. The next most powerful variables were the interaction between nonbinary responses and accessibility and the interaction between nonbinary questions and positive social desirability.

Because of the large number of significant interaction effects in this model, an understanding of the effect on response accuracy of the significant variables can best be achieved by considering main effects along with any associated interactions. Four clusters of variables thus formed will now be discussed.

The first cluster consisted of accessibility, response type, and their interaction. By themselves, accessibility had a positive association with response accuracy, and binary questions were more accurate than nonbinary questions. The significant negative interaction between the variables, however, suggests that when the information requested in a survey was relatively inaccessible, greater response accuracy was obtained when the response called for was other than a simple yes or no. Put another way, accessibility had a greater impact on binary questions. Binary, accessible questions tended to have the highest rates of response accuracy, while questions that were binary and inaccessible tended to have the lowest rates.

Response type, positive social desirability, and their interaction comprised the second group of variables. Again, binary questions were more accurate than nonbinary questions. The positive main effect for positive social desirability and the lack of a significant main effect for negative social desirability questions suggest that positive social desirability questions were more accurate than questions in the indeterminate and negative categories, other things being equal. However, as indicated by the interaction, the negative effect of being nonbinary was heightened for positive socially desirable response direction questions. That binary questions to which the socially desirable response was positive were more accurate may simply reflect the fact that all of the respondents had participated in the behavior, thereby eliminating the possibility of false positive replies. On the other hand, for questions concerning socially desirable behaviors to which responses are nonbinary, respondents may tend to exaggerate claims.

The third variable cluster consisted of accessibility, positive social desirability, and the interaction between accessibility and both of the dummy variables representing socially desirable response direction. As previously discussed, both accessibility and positive social desirability were positively associated with response accuracy. Significant interaction effects between both of the dummy variables for socially desirable response direction and accessibility, however, indicate that the effect of accessibility on response accuracy was strongest for questions in the indeterminate response direction category. There was not a significant main effect for negative social desirability, so the negative coefficient for its interaction with accessibility suggests that the effect of negative social desirability, at least relative to the indeterminate category, is very much dependent upon the accessibility of the information.

These findings are difficult to interpret because questions were categorized as indeterminate for different reasons, including when the socially desirable response direction was positive for some respondents, but negative for others; unclear; or an irrelevant issue. However, it makes sense that when the information requested is accessible and the response is socially neutral, accuracy would be high.

The fourth group of variables included positive social desirability and its interaction with the questionnaire method. As already noted, questions that were classified as having a positive socially desirable response direction tended to be more accurate than questions categorized as negative or indeterminate. Further, positive socially desirable response direction items that were presented to respondents in a questionnaire were more accurate than those asked in a face-to-face interview.

Because all of the respondents for these reverse record check sample questions possessed the item in question or had participated in the behavior, false positive responses were not possible. Distortions of amounts in responses to nonbinary questions, however, could have occurred. In fact, there were only three questions that were categorized as positive socially desirable response direction questionnaire items for this reverse record check sample subset, and all three were nonbinary. These were two questions concerning the number of Union Leadership classes attended and one question about current gross salary. In contrast, there were 33 positive socially desirable response direction face-to-face interview items, both binary and nonbinary, largely concerning savings account ownership and size. Any interpretations of our findings must take into consideration this dissimilarity across categories in item response type and content. Perhaps exaggeration in response to nonbinary questions was minimized on a questionnaire as opposed to in a face-to-face interview, because the latter may increase the salience of social desirability concerns, thereby encouraging this exaggeration. Questionnaires may also provide an opportunity to think through a response or to consult records or other people. It is also possible, however, that certain types of questions, for example, concerning savings account amounts, were more susceptible to response distortion.

Concerning question type, responses to deviant questions were more accurate than responses to descriptive information and behavior or financial matters questions. In part, this finding may be attributable to high levels of inaccuracy in responses to the large number of financial matters questions included in this reverse record check question subset. In the weighted analyses of general sample questions, financial matters questions represented, in both cases, only about 7% of the total group of questions. However, in the weighted analysis of the reverse record check sample questions, financial questions amounted to about 65% of the total. Further, there were about five times as many financial matters questions as there were descriptive information and behavior questions. Considered in this light, the interpretation of this finding may be that exaggerations, minimizations, or denials are more likely in response to financial matters questions than to questions concerning deviant and personal behavior.

Finally, the significant main effect for study date indicated that questions from earlier studies tended to be more accurate than questions from more recent studies.

10

Meta-Analysis: Discussion and Integration

In order to draw any overall conclusions concerning the relationship between survey question characteristics and response accuracy for the questions included in this investigation, the separate meta-analyses findings must be compared and possibly integrated. In this effort, it is important to recall that the particular variables included in each of the three regression analyses differed slightly, largely because of differences in the numbers of questions in the categories of the discrete variables for the three question groups. Thus, the factor/factor interactions which were included for analysis in one case could not be evaluated in another. Also, socially desirable response direction was a two-category variable in the two general sample question group analyses, but a three-category variable in the analysis of the reverse record check sample questions.

In these exploratory analyses, we sought to examine as many question characteristics as possible and, therefore, included variables in an analysis whenever we could. We are aware that some loss may have resulted in terms of the strict comparability of the findings of the three analyses. We also believe, however, that any potential loss is more than compensated for by the gain in the form of increased understanding of the effect on response accuracy of particular question attributes, including those resulting from variable interactions. Considering the analyses results, the importance of interaction effects on the regression models is obvious.

Because the group of general sample questions which included the prevalence variable is a subset of the larger group of general sample questions, a comparison will first be made between the regression analyses results for those two question groups. Next, we will compare regression analyses results for general and reverse record check sample questions. In this latter comparison, we are interested in determining whether the variables associated with response accuracy are the same or different for the two sample types. Possibly, respondents who have all performed a behavior react differently as a group to survey question attributes than a respondent group which includes both performers and nonperformers.

General Sample Questions Analyses

Similarities between the analyses performed on the two general sample question groups was expected and obtained. The inclusion of the prevalence variable in the second analysis, however, allowed for an examination of the effects on response accuracy of behavioral prevalence, both in and of itself and in interaction with other variables. Important information was also gleaned from the analysis results for the total group of general sample questions, because the increased number of questions in that group allowed for the inclusion of more interactions and also, perhaps, allowed for more confidence in certain outcomes.

In both analyses, response accuracy was greater for questions where the information requested was accessible and the study date was relatively recent. Also, responses to questions for which the socially desirable response was positive were *less* accurate than responses to negative socially desirable response direction questions. Further, increased sensitivity was in general related to decreased accuracy.

Response type, included in both analyses, was significant only in the regression analysis for the total group of general sample questions, as a main effect and also in interaction with question sensitivity. For this group, binary questions tended to be more accurate than nonbinary questions. Further, the interaction effect signifies that respondents answered particularly sensitive questions more truthfully when the response called for was other than a simple "yes" or "no." We tend to accept these findings as applicable to all general sample questions because, in these weighted analyses, the question subset with prevalence information contained 65 binary questions but only 3 nonbinary questions, which may be an insufficient number for a valid comparison. In contrast, the larger general sample question group, although still containing mainly binary questions, also consisted of 12 nonbinary questions.

In the question subset with prevalence information, prevalence had a significant main effect and also was significant in interaction with deviant/personal questions. As discussed in connection with the second analysis, the progress of the regression analyses results for the prevalence subset with respect to the question type variable paralleled the results for the total group of general sample questions until the interaction between prevalence and deviant/personal question type was included. Therefore, we conclude that these findings from the prevalence subset pertain to all general sample questions. To summarize, of the question type categories, descriptive information and behavior questions tended to be the most accurate, followed by financial matters questions. For those question types, prevalence and accuracy were positively associated. For the least accurate deviant and personal behavior questions, greater accuracy was related to lower behavioral prevalence.

More accurate responses to questions on deviant and personal behavior were obtained with questionnaires than in face-to-face interviews. Although method by itself was insignificant in both analyses, in the analysis of the total group of general sample questions, there was a significant interaction between method and deviant/personal questions. For the general sample questions with prevalence information, there was an insufficient number of questions to include that interaction in the regression analysis.

In this comparison and integration of the regression analysis results for the two general sample groups, 11 variables in all were significant. The variation in percentage of accurate responses accounted for by the 10 significant variables in the analysis of the total group of general sample questions was 66%, and 84% by the 8 significant variables in the prevalence subset.

General and Reverse Record Check Samples Analyses

A comparison between the results for the reverse record check sample questions and the summarized results for the general sample questions reveals many similarities, but also important differences. For example, interaction effects were more prominent in the reverse record check sample questions analysis than in the general sample questions analysis. Many of these differences were not explicable except by reference to the essential dissimilarity between the two sample types, namely, the difference in behavioral prevalence. For general samples the percentages of performers varied, while for reverse record check samples all of the respondents were performers. This difference in the composition of the respondent groups apparently resulted in certain differences both in the variables associated with response accuracy and in the direction of the associations. Our decision to separate the groups for analysis is supported by the fact of different findings.

For both sample types, accessibility had a significant positive effect on response accuracy, and binary questions were responded to more accurately than nonbinary questions. However, for reverse record check sample questions only, accessibility and response type also significantly interacted. That is, for the reverse record check sample questions, when requested information was relatively inaccessible, more truthful replies were obtained if the questions were posed in a nonbinary format. For these nonbinary questions, respondents' recall may have been assisted by the provision of response categories, or more simply, by the necessity to think through a response as opposed to just offering a yes or no answer.[1] That this significant interaction effect was *not* found in the analyses of general sample questions may be due to the possibility that there were not enough nonbinary, inaccessible questions included in the general sample analyses for the effect to emerge (see Table 8.5). For the reverse record check sample questions, nonbinary questions represented about 65% of the weighted total, as opposed to less than 9% of the weighted total in the groups of general sample questions.

Sensitivity was a significant variable only in the general sample questions analyses, with sensitivity and accuracy being inversely related. However, we tend to conclude that sensitivity is in general an important variable affecting response accuracy. Since values for this variable were obtained from raters, we thought that perhaps we had not judged sensitivity as well for the performers-only samples.

Alternatively, the failure of question sensitivity to significantly affect response accuracy for the reverse record check sample questions may perhaps again be attributable to the somewhat different characteristics of the particular questions included in the two sample types. For example, the reverse record check sample set contained a large percentage of financial matters questions—about 65% of the weighted total as opposed to approximately 7% of the weighted total for the general sample sets. Questions about financial matters are likely not only sensitive, but if often calling for a nonbinary response, also comparatively inaccessible. In reviewing the intercorrelations for the reverse record check sample questions among the four variables—sensitivity, accessibility, response type, and question type—just such a picture emerges (see footnote 21 in Chapter 8). This pattern of interrelationships, which is different in certain cases from the pattern for the general sample questions, and which possibly reflects the overrepresentation of financial matters questions in this reverse record check group, may have resulted in the failure to find a main effect for sensitivity.

A significant interaction between sensitivity and response type was found only for the general sample questions, perhaps because, as discussed previously, the sensitivity variable was insignificant in the reverse record check sample questions analysis. The interpretation of this interaction was that particularly sensitive questions were responded to more truthfully when the response called for was other than a simple yes or no.

---

[1]Since complete descriptions of the questions analyzed in this report were often not provided, it is not possible to determine with certainty in which cases categories were or were not provided for respondents.

In an effort to understand why this would be so, we examined the general sample questions for instances of sensitive, nonbinary items. Apparently, a large number of these questions concerned socially undesirable events or behavior; for example, arrests or the performance of deviant or illegal acts such as theft. Phrased to elicit a binary response, these questions might simply have asked, "Have you ever....?" and been met by predictable denials. However, a nonbinary question commonly asks, "How often have you...?" The latter type question seems to have two implications. The first is that the respondent has performed the behavior, at least once. If there is no filter question, the second implication is that the behavior is prevalent and perhaps, therefore, not so deviant after all. All that needs to be established is frequency. If the respondent makes the corresponding inferences, the result is a desensitization of the topic and an increase in accuracy.

As we have previously noted, the questions included in these analyses did not necessarily make for a balanced design.[2] Certain question dimensions, or variable categories, were better represented than others. The fact that sensitive, nonbinary, general sample questions tended to concern socially undesirable behavior is an example of what may be thought of as a design problem or limitation.

For general samples, positive socially desirable response direction questions were responded to *less* accurately than negative direction questions. In the reverse record check sample questions analysis, positive socially desirable response direction questions tended to be *more* accurate than negative or indeterminate direction questions. These discrepant findings, however, are reconcilable when we interpret the general sample results as suggesting that false claims of socially desirable behavior are more likely than either untruthful denials or false claims of socially undesirable behavior.[3] In other words, respondents wish to claim, and rarely deny, performance of socially desirable acts. Therefore, when positive socially desirable response direction questions were directed to samples where all respondents had actually engaged in the behavior, so that false positive replies were not possible, the predictable result was a high rate of accuracy. Behavior that was not socially desirable was, in contrast, more frequently denied; false claims again were not possible in these questions. Overall, then, we tend to conclude that for items where the socially desirable response is positive, and when the sample is constituted such that false claims are possible, these false claims of socially desirable behavior will tend to occur more

---

[2] See Chapter 8, footnote 20.

[3] Refer to the discussion of the socially desirable response direction variable in Chapter 8. False claims or exaggerations of socially undesirable behavior were not unusual in these data.

frequently than untruthful denials or false claims of socially undesirable behavior.

This interpretation is supported by the significant negative interaction found in the reverse record check sample questions analysis between response type and the dummy variable representing the comparison between positive socially desirable response direction items and all other questions, including both those for which the socially desirable response was to say "no" and those classified as indeterminate. In this analysis, as expected, those positive socially desirable behavior items posed in a nonbinary format were less accurate than those positive items calling simply for either a yes or no response — a finding that is simply artifactual due to the nature of a reverse record check sample. Further, exaggerations of positive behavior were apparently again more common than minimizations or exaggerations of socially undesirable or indeterminate behavior. On the other hand, negative or indeterminate social desirability items were more accurate when presented in a nonbinary as opposed to a binary format. Since indeterminate items swamped negative socially desirable direction items — 29 versus 13 in the weighted analysis — this finding is difficult to interpret. Considering just the negative category, it appears that minimizations or exaggerations of socially disapproved behavior are less likely than outright denials.

We tend to accept this finding as applying to both sample types. The specific interaction could not be tested in the general sample questions analyses due to an insufficient number of cases in certain cells of the factor/factor interaction. However, the result is consistent with the finding and related interpretation for the general sample items, discussed previously, concerning the interaction between sensitivity and response type.

When the indeterminate category for socially desirable response direction was included in the reverse record check questions analysis, significant negative interactions resulted between accessibility and both of the dummy variables representing socially desirable response direction. This finding indicates that accessibility had the greatest impact on questions for which the direction of the socially desirable response was classified as indeterminate, that is, either positive for some respondents but negative for others, or unclear, or an irrelevant issue. Further, this impact was especially pronounced when the information requested was relatively inaccessible. Since, due to an insufficient number of questions, the indeterminate category was not included in the analyses of the general sample questions, we tend to accept the above finding as applying to both sample types.

The interpretation of these interactions is difficult because of the different bases for classifying questions in the indeterminate category. That socially neutral, accessible information would be reported quite accurately, however, seems reasonable. We might also expect that for inaccessible information, as opposed to having a negative or positive socially desirable response direction, that which is also socially neutral would be the least accurate. That is, socially neutral, inaccessible information may be the most difficult to recall because it is not associated in memory with attitudes or opinions concerning social desirability and, perhaps by extension, with individuals' beliefs about themselves.

Although not significant as a main effect in any of the analyses, method was significant in interaction, but with a different variable for each sample type. In the reverse record check sample questions analysis, we found a significant positive interaction between method and the dummy variable comparing those questions to which the socially desirable response was positive to all other questions. As discussed above, this interaction apparently signified that, concerning items for which the socially desirable response was positive, respondents provided more truthful replies—that is, in this case, they exaggerated less—when these items were presented in a questionnaire as opposed to a face-to-face interview. Perhaps self-presentational and social approval issues are less salient in a questionnaire situation, so that respondents are less likely to exaggerate claims of socially desirable behavior. Questionnaires may also provide respondents with opportunities to consult records or other people and more time to think through a response.

On the other hand, for questions where either social desirability was not able to be determined, or for which the socially desirable response was to say no or to minimize, greater accuracy was generally obtained with face-to-face interviews than with questionnaires. Because of the many reasons for classifying a question as indeterminate, this finding is difficult to interpret. However, social neutrality was one of the reasons, and indeterminate questions outnumbered negative social desirability items in the weighted analysis by about 3 to 1. Perhaps socially neutral information, which may not be readily accessible to memory, is more easily remembered in a face-to-face situation than on a questionnaire because an interviewer may use probes to assist recall. Further, the motivation to be a "good subject" is probably heightened in a face-to-face situation. When social desirability and self-presentation are not issues, this motivation may also lead to more accurate responding.

The significant interaction between method and positive social desirability found in the reverse record check sample questions analysis appears to be attributable to the presence of this group of indeterminate questions and also to the fact that all positive socially desirable response direction question items coincidentally were also nonbinary. When the indeterminate category was not represented at all in the general sample questions analyses due to an insufficient number of cases, the interaction between method and socially desirable response direction was insignificant. An exact comparison between the findings for the two sample types is limited by these dissimilarities, especially in the categories included in the socially desirable response direction variable. We tend to accept the findings from the reverse record check analysis in this regard, however, because the inclusion for evaluation of social neutrality — apparently a true characteristic of certain questions — makes the reverse record check analysis more complete.

The significant interaction between method and one of the dummy variables for question type in the analysis of all general sample questions indicated that for deviant and personal behavior questions, more accurate responses were obtained with questionnaires than in face-to-face interviews. The deviant and personal behavior items included in the general sample questions tended to be nonbinary. As we have already noted, nonbinary questions appear to be answered more truthfully on questionnaires. Possible explanations include that more time is allowed to think through a response, categories may be available which assist recall, or an opportunity to consult other people or records is provided. This factor/factor interaction could not be tested in the reverse record check sample questions analysis because of an insufficient number of cases in certain cells when the variables were cross-tabulated. This finding, however, is consistent with other findings and related interpretations for the reverse record check sample, for example, concerning the interaction between method and socially desirable response direction.

We expected that descriptive information and behavior questions would be responded to more accurately overall than either deviant and personal behavior or financial matters questions. Although this expectation was supported by the findings for the general sample questions with financial matters questions generally intermediate in accuracy levels, the highest percentages of accuracy for reverse record check samples tended to occur for questions in the deviant category.

The fact that there are different sources of error for the two sample types fails to explain these contrary findings. That is, false claims are not possible in reverse record check samples. If false claims were a larger source of error in responses to deviant and personal behavior questions than in responses to the other question types, then removing that source of error might result in a comparatively high overall level of response accuracy for those deviant and personal behavior questions. However, when false claims were possible, as in general sample questions, then deviant and personal behavior questions would tend to have comparatively low accuracy levels.

We know from the above discussion of the socially desirable response direction variable that false claims of undesirable behavior do occur. However, we need to determine the extent of this type of error in the various question categories. Although they include only an unrepresentative portion of the total number of questions included in this study and are limited also to only binary questions, the data in Table 7.1 lend themselves to an examination of sources of error by question type, and therefore are at least suggestive of the distribution of this error. Looking at the general sample questions only, we compared the percentages of respondents who denied the behavior with the percentages who made false claims. The resulting unweighted mean percentages for the three question categories were about 1.5% versus 13.6% for the descriptive information and behavior questions ($N = 18$), 8.2% versus 4.8% for the deviant and personal behavior questions ($N = 6$), and 11% versus 13.2% for the financial matters questions ($N = 4$). From this data, it appears that while false claims of deviant and personal behavior do occur, this source of error is least common in that question category.

A second possible explanation for the contrary findings is that even within the same question type categories, the particular questions addressed to respondents in the reverse record check samples may have coincidentally differed from those addressed to general sample respondents along some underlying dimension or dimensions associated with response accuracy and perhaps not measured in this study. Even considering the variables that we did measure, the pattern of interrelationships was somewhat different for the two sample types. This would account for the instability in the relative accuracy of the question type categories from one analysis to another, especially considering that differences in relative accuracy were probably, even initially, not very great (see Table 8.4).

Further, this explanation suggests that while it is commonly believed that question type is a central variable affecting survey response validity, in fact, question type in and of itself may be relatively unimportant in predicting response accuracy.

Included only in the analysis of a general sample questions subset, prevalence was significantly associated with response accuracy and also interacted with question type. For both descriptive information and behavior and financial matters questions, prevalence was positively associated with accuracy. For deviant questions, however, the association between prevalence and response accuracy was reversed.

Regarding study date, accuracy tended to increase over time for general sample questions but decrease for reverse record check sample questions. One possible explanation for these discrepant findings is suggested by the weighted frequency distribution of the 78 reverse record check cases by study date. In the time span from 1970 on, there is only 1 question; in the time span from 1960 to 1970, there are 22 questions. The bulk of the reverse record check sample questions, then, about 71%, were taken from pre-1960 surveys. In sharp contrast, although 42% of the general sample questions are also pre-1960, a full 40% are post-1970. The relatively small number of reverse record check sample questions from recent years may have resulted in an inadequate assessment of the relationship between study date and response accuracy for that group.

11

Meta-Analysis: Summary and Conclusions

Having described, discussed, and integrated the results of the three meta-analyses, we will now attempt to summarize our findings and to draw certain specific conclusions about the relationship between survey question characteristics and response accuracy.

Looking at the results in a general way, it is apparent that the main effects measured and included in these analyses have been quite potent in explaining response accuracy, since all but two were significant in the regression models. Sensitivity was significant only in the general sample questions analyses. Method was insignificant for both sample types. Judging from the high percentages of variation in response accuracy explained by the variables we have measured in this investigation, we conclude that we have in fact identified key survey question characteristics affecting respondents' reports.

That method was insignificant as a main effect in all three regression models is itself of interest since method is among the variables commonly believed to impact response validity. In our analysis, we included method and other frequently discussed variables such as question sensitivity and question type. However, we also considered additional characteristics, such as response type, accessibility, and the direction of the socially desirable response. Further, in our systematic analyses, we included these variables not only as main effects, but in interaction with other variables. That interaction effects were prominent in our results demonstrates the complexity of the relationship between question attributes and response accuracy.

Accessibility, Response Type, and Their Interaction

Looking at the results in particular, the dominant variable was accessibility, or the availability to recall of the requested information. If the information requested had been judged to be comparatively easy to remember, then replies were more accurate. Accessibility also interacted with other variables, including response type.

Overall, questions which called for a simple "yes" or "no" response were more accurate than those that required a nonbinary response, such as the specification of an amount or a frequency. This makes sense because nonbinary questions ask for more information, and specifications might be hard to remember. We know, however, that for many reasons, interviewees will offer a response, even if they are uncertain. These reasons include trying to please the interviewer and not wishing to appear uncooperative, uninformed, or unaware (Sudman & Bradburn, 1974).

When the information requested, however, was judged to be relatively inaccessible, more truthful replies were obtained to nonbinary than to binary questions. We reasoned that, with nonbinary questions, the categories that are sometimes provided might prompt associations, thereby aiding recall. On the other hand, categories may encourage premature closure if respondents focus outward on the choices, perhaps thinking of them as self-descriptions, as opposed to focusing inward and engaging in a memory search.

Other possible problems with the use of categories were discussed at length in Chapter 6. These problems include the possible operation of the anchoring effect. Also, when categories are provided and the information requested is relatively inaccessible, respondents may be more likely to select an approximation from the choices presented, as opposed to attempting to retrieve and locate the precisely correct response.

Unfortunately, the comparative accuracy of responses to questions calling for a nonbinary response where categories were or were not provided cannot be ascertained with our data. As noted in Chapter 10, footnote 1, we were not always able to determine from the information provided in the studies included in our analysis when categories had in fact been used. Further investigation in this area is needed.

The use of categories, however, appears to introduce a number of potential problems that would result in decreased response accuracy, perhaps especially when the information is inaccessible. As another possible explanation for the finding that questions about inaccessible information were responded to *more* accurately when these type questions were presented in a nonbinary format, we suspect that respondents answer binary questions more quickly than nonbinary questions, again to avoid appearing uninformed, uncooperative, or unaware. On the other hand, pauses, or taking time to reflect, are probably viewed as acceptable in response to nonbinary questions. In responding to questions where the information requested is relatively inaccessible, greater accuracy may then result from taking this additional time to retrieve information.

That time to respond and response accuracy are related is also suggested by our data at several other points, and will be discussed at length in a later section. Based on our findings, we conclude that spending time on a question appears to be related to increased response accuracy. Importantly, we are now able to specify certain conditions under which respondents apparently need this additional time — in this case, to retrieve comparatively inaccessible information. As detailed in Chapter 6, there is strong theoretical and research support in the cognitive psychology literature for this interpretation.

Our research also enables us, here and in other instances to be discussed, to specify particular methods that can be used in attempts to increase the validity of survey responses. For example, when information is judged to be relatively inaccessible, our data suggest that more positive results would be obtained by posing questions in a nonbinary format, probably not involving the use of categories.[1] That this increased accuracy is attributable to the fact that nonbinary questions provide a situation where respondents take more time to answer than they do when asked a binary question is a possibility that needs further direct investigation.

Accessibility was the most potent variable in our analysis. In our discussion about the effects of accessibility on response accuracy, we have focused on inaccessible questions because these were problematic in terms of response accuracy. We should not forget, however, that information judged to be accessible tended to be reported accurately, suggesting that respondents will be truthful if they can. Considerations apparently affecting their ability and inclination to be truthful include whether the information is or is judged to be available in memory (Tulving & Pearlstone, 1966); the amount of access time needed as compared with the amount of time actually or perceived to be

---

[1]It is important to recall that accessibility and accuracy were related as expected in our analyses. Apparently, then, we were able to generally make accurate judgments concerning the accessibility of the information requested in the survey questions included in our study—that is, accurate judgments about the type of autobiographical information that people in general have difficulty remembering. Importantly, in contrast to the feeling-of-knowing methodology used in research on cognitive processes (e.g., Yaniv & Meyer, 1987), where individuals provide self-ratings concerning the accessibility of particular information, with our procedure we made apparently valid accessibility judgments *for others*.

Some additional support for our method of rating accessibility for others comes from research on the subject of eyewitness identification. It seems reasonable to suppose that the degree of confidence expressed by eyewitnesses in their judgments would be related to identification accuracy. In fact, however, the confidence–accuracy relationship has been found to be extremely variable and, on the average, negligible (Cutler *et al.*, 1987). Individuals who are aware of factors that may have influenced encoding and that may affect retrieval may, in fact, be in a better position to make judgments about the likelihood of eyewitness identification accuracy or, put another way, about accessibility.

available; the costs associated with recall attempts, for example, in terms of effort; and perhaps the benefits associated with accuracy.

The above interpretation suggests ways to increase the accuracy of reports of available but inaccessible information. These include providing respondents with more retrieval time, through, for example, the use of nonbinary questions; increasing the motivation to expend time and effort, perhaps through providing appropriate recall conditions or through increasing the obtained benefits (payments to respondents, promises of feedback, and attempts to stress the importance of participation are perhaps examples of this); and/or reducing time and effort expenditures through providing optimal recall conditions.

Concerning the second option, Hasher & Griffin (1978) hypothesized that increased effort induced by certain procedures used in their research on the recall of prose passages may have been the factor responsible for greater accuracy of recall in those conditions.

With respect to the last option, the amount of time and effort necessary to retrieve requested information may be decreased if certain factors are considered when survey questions are crafted and instruments are developed. That the use of appropriate cues, probes, or context can prompt the choice of appropriate and effective response strategies, facilitate the retrieval process, and contribute to response accuracy is strongly supported in the literature (see our discussion of this subject in Chapter 6). In our research, we were not able to evaluate these factors because information on exact question wording and on question order, or context, was often not available in the published reports.

Question Sensitivity and Response Type

Returning to our specific findings, response type also interacted with sensitivity. By itself, as expected, sensitivity had a negative association with response accuracy. Concerning particularly sensitive questions, as with questions about relatively inaccessible information, respondents were more truthful when the response called for was other than a simple "yes" or "no." We suspected that when questions ask for an amount or frequency, and if there is no filter question, there are two implications. The first implication is that the respondent has performed the behavior at least once. Second, the behavior may be more prevalent than the respondent believed. The result is that the topic is somewhat desensitized.

We recall our speculation that nonbinary questions also permit the respondent to take more time to answer. With binary questions, respondents may believe that hesitation concerning sensitive topics would be viewed by the interviewer as defensive behavior, with the respondent being uncomfortable and having something to hide. With nonbinary questions, taking time — pausing — is acceptable. As with inaccessible information, this time may be useful to retrieve the specific information requested, as opposed to, in the case of sensitive questions, providing a response based on social desirability or self-presentation concerns or, indeed, denial.[2]

Direction of the Socially Desirable Response

Turning to the matter of the direction of the socially desirable response, we found that responses to questions for which the socially desirable response was to say "yes" or to exaggerate were *less* accurate than responses to negative socially desirable response direction questions. In other words, false claims or exaggerations of socially desirable behavior occur more frequently than untruthful denials, false claims, minimizations, or exaggerations of socially undesirable behavior. We suspect that this result cannot be fully explained as a simple misrepresentation of the facts by respondents. If that were the case, it would be reasonable to expect that subjects' motivation to exaggerate the positive would be similar to their motivation to minimize the negative.

A more satisfactory explanation for our results is provided by certain theories and research in the area of cognitive organization and processes, especially with respect to the concept of schemas. Briefly defined, schemas are "structures which encode and represent knowledge" (Markus, 1980, p. 106) and are similar to the concepts of knowledge structures or scripts discussed in Chapter 6. According to Markus (1980), self-schemas contain ideas about the self and, in the interests of efficiency of information processing and ease of retrieval, may tend more toward generalizations or summaries as we develop. Very general schemas about the self "come from the repeated similar categorizations of the self across many different situations" (Markus, 1980, p. 113).

---

[2]This interpretation may explain the failure to find a significant main effect for sensitivity in the reverse record check questions analysis. In the intercorrelation matrix, the relationship between accessibility and sensitivity was significant for both the general sample and the reverse record check sample questions. However, the direction of the association was different for the two groups. In the case of the general sample questions the relationship was positive. In other words, questions which were rated as comparatively accessible were also viewed as being relatively sensitive, while inaccessible questions tended not to be sensitive. For reverse record check questions, the reverse was true. Therefore, inaccessibility and sensitivity were characteristics of the same questions. Since accessibility was the dominant variable in terms of its association with accuracy, its inclusion in the regression equation washed out the effect of sensitivity.

Let us examine the concept of schemas as it helps us understand the tendency of respondents to exaggerate their performance of socially desirable behavior and to minimize or deny their performance of socially undesirable behavior.

Exaggerated Performance of Socially Desirable Behavior

That we tend to perceive ourselves favorably is supported by research in social psychology, for example, on the self-serving bias and on the tendency of individuals to view themselves as being "better than average" (e.g., Myers & Ridl, 1979, p. 89). General self-schemas, then, would tend to be positive self-descriptions. If subjects consult these general schemas when they respond to survey questions, their responses will indicate performance, or exaggerated performance, of socially desirable activities.

The above explanation is consistent with Cahalan's (1968) reasoning that individuals' responses may sometimes be based on knowledge about what they usually do or on what they should have done, rather than on what they actually did. For example, individuals may have a "good citizen" self-schema, based on fairly regular voting behavior. When asked about voting in a particular election, subjects may refer to this schema and conclude that because they are good citizens who usually vote, they must have voted in that election.

Theoretical support for the existence of bias in autobiographical memories may be found in the work of Tulving (1985), who proposed the existence of three major memory systems. Knowledge about personally experienced events was associated with the episodic memory system. According to Tulving, representations in episodic memory involve the individual's personal identity. Episodic memory is characterized by "autonoetic (self-knowing) consciousness" (p. 388) that

> ... allows an individual to become aware of his or her own identity
> and existence in subjective time that extends from the past through
> the present to the future. It provides the familiar phenomenal
> flavor of recollective experience characterized by "pastness" and
> *subjective veridicality*. [Tulving, 1985, p. 388, emphasis added]

Effect of Method on Tendency to Exaggerate
Research by Markus (1980) suggests that information that is inconsistent with self-schemas may take longer to process. We have already demonstrated that time may be necessary to access certain kinds of information. Information about occasions when respondents failed to act consistently with self-schemas, that is failed to act in socially desirable or positive ways,

may also take more time to access. This possibility is supported by our finding that there was less exaggeration in response to positive socially desirable response direction questions on questionnaires than in face-to-face interviews.

That there are differences in accuracy levels depending on the method used also supports our conclusion that respondents are not always misrepresenting facts. If so, the tendency to be untruthful should reveal itself irrespective of the data-gathering method. What we seem to be finding instead is that certain conditions assist respondents' recall of information, or decrease the probability of error. For questions about socially desirable events, respondents may need time to reflect about particular behaviors. Questionnaires may provide this additional response time.

Concerns about self-presentation and social approval may also be less prominent in a questionnaire situation. In other words, the presence of an interviewer may heighten the saliency of social or normative expectations. The response strategy chosen, then, may tend to reflect social desirability concerns as opposed to concerns with specific information retrieval.

That the presence of others influences behavior has been demonstrated in social psychological research, for example, in the studies on bystander intervention (e.g., Latane & Darley, 1970) and on the social facilitation effect (e.g., Zajonc, 1965). That the presence of others specifically motivates responses that are perceived to be socially desirable is supported in Asch's classic studies on conformity (Asch, 1951). When allowed to write their answers, as opposed to responding publicly, Asch's subjects were less influenced by group pressure, that is, were less likely to make judgments indicating conformity (Myers, 1990).

In his research on obedience to authority, Milgram (1974) found that the physical presence of the authority figure affected the level of obedience. When the subject was not under the surveillance of the experimenter, the level of obedience dropped. Perhaps in the presence of the experimenter, subjects' concerns were focused on perceived social expectations or on the norms governing superior–subordinate relationships. When alone, subjects may have been less affected by social desirability concerns because they may have been more self-focused, that is, focused on their inner dispositions and attitudes toward this particular task. Research supports that increasing the level of self-consciousness or self-awareness affects behavior (Diener & Wallbom, 1976).

Milgram's data is additionally relevant in the context of survey research because the social influence effects that Milgram observed occurred in a situation where there were clear status differences between the subject and the experimenter. In those cases, social influence effects may be especially great. The survey interview situation is one in which status differences are likely to be perceived. Research indicates that just because they ask the questions, interviewers will be perceived as more knowledgeable than interviewees (Ross, Amabile, & Steinmetz, 1977).

Another possible explanation for the superiority of questionnaires for positive socially desirable response direction questions is that questionnaires may allow respondents to concentrate more fully on the question content. Perhaps seeing the words keeps respondents' attention focused on the question longer than simply hearing the words. The question context is also evident and may provide important cues for recall. Energies are focused on the question itself and on the retrieval of the requested information, and perhaps less, then, on self-presentational or social desirability concerns.

In this regard, Baddeley, Lewis, Eldridge, & Thomson (1984) found that subjects' productivity was negatively affected when they were required to listen to and repeat digits while generating items from given categories. Perhaps concerns or distractions occasioned by the presence of an interviewer act as a competing task which affects retrieval. Referring back to the description of long-term memory offered by Ericsson & Simon (1980) and presented in Chapter 6, the authors stated that short-term memory may be used to store intermediate steps in the retrieval process. The presentation of competing or distracting information may disrupt this process by intruding on short-term memory stores. In the case of surveys, unlike in Baddeley *et al.*'s study, the disruption may be great because the competing task is directly related to the task at hand. That is, the presence of an interviewer may create a situation where respondents must choose among such alternative concerns as self-presentation, social desirability responding, or truthful reply. Inaccurate responses may then often result.

If questionnaires are left with the respondent, they also afford an opportunity to consult records or other people. Whatever the specific explanation may be, it nevertheless appears that the tendency on the part of respondents to enhance their self-descriptions may be able to be counteracted by using questionnaires to obtain information on socially desirable events or behaviors.

Denials or Minimizations of Undesirable Behavior

The tendency of respondents to minimize the negative also needs explanation. The performance of unusual behaviors, for example, socially undesirable behaviors, may be inconsistent with self-schemas and, therefore, less accessible. When asked about performance of socially undesirable behaviors, subjects may refer to these self-schemas and then make inferences concerning their behavior. Cahalan (1968) expressed this possibility as follows:

> If the question permits the respondent to misinterpret or re-
> construct his memories so he can give a response that is more
> congruent with his own self-respect than the actual facts would
> be, he may tend to rewrite history more in line with what he
> thinks he ought to have done than with what he actually did.
> [pp. 609–610]

Other researchers have also expressed the belief that individuals sometimes construct or reconstruct their memories in a positive direction. In
other words, at least concerning certain types of issues, they may not be
telling the truth to themselves (e.g., Loftus *et al.*, 1985; Markus, 1980).

There is support for the idea that current beliefs about the self affect the
recall of past self-referent information. For example, researchers found that
subjects' reports of past attitudes were that they were identical with current
attitudes, even when the current attitude was clearly different from the one
expressed earlier, and even when researchers told the subjects that they
were in possession of the subjects' original attitude statements and that the accuracy of their recall could be checked (Nisbett & Wilson, 1977). Further, as
reported in Chapter 4, Robins (1966) found that subjects who had been arrested in the past were more likely to report this if their arrest histories
continued into the present or, in other words, if their past and present behaviors were consistent.

Lack of spontaneous rehearsal (see, e.g., Banaji & Crowder, 1989) may
account for the difficulty in retrieving memories of socially disapproved behavior. Rehearsal of behavior that is inconsistent with self-schemas might
occasion negative self-evaluations. Lack of rehearsal is also believed to be one
of the mechanisms through which repression is accomplished (Erdelyi, in
press, as cited in Banaji & Crowder, 1989).

Effect of Response Type on Tendency to Minimize

As with inaccessible or very sensitive question topics, we found that when the
socially desirable response was to say "no" or to minimize, obtained responses were more accurate when the questions were posed in a nonbinary
as opposed to a binary format. That is, minimizations or exaggerations of
socially disapproved behavior were less likely than outright denials. Our
interpretation is consistent with conclusions we have drawn from other findings. In the case of socially disapproved behavior, as with highly sensitive
questions, asking about frequency may suggest that the respondent and also
other individuals have in fact engaged in the behavior. This may reduce the
likelihood that the behavior will be perceived as socially undesirable or
deviant, which may, in turn, reduce the amount of social desirability responding. Also, as previously discussed, nonbinary questions may allow a respondent time to reflect.

Why Tendency to Exaggerate the Positive Is Greater Than Tendency to Minimize the Negative

We have attempted to provide explanations for our findings that respondents sometimes exaggerate performance of socially desirable behaviors and minimize performance of socially undesirable behaviors. Recall, however, that reports about socially undesirable behavior were *more* accurate than reports about socially desirable behavior. As opposed to failure actions, that is, failures to behave in socially desirable ways, perhaps instances of actually performing socially undesirable behavior are more distinct in an individual's life and, as such, are more accessible to recall. As an extreme example of the effect of distinctiveness on recall, researchers (e.g., Brown, 1986) use the term "flashbulb memory" (p. 270) to refer to the very vivid recollections individuals have of certain very unique and spectacular events in their lives.

Reports of Socially Neutral Information Affected by Method and Accessibility

Concerning questions which were judged to be either indeterminate or neutral in terms of the direction of the socially desirable response, greater accuracy was obtained in face-to-face interviews than through questionnaires. In the case of socially neutral information, we concluded that recall of this type of information may be assisted by the probes of skillful interviewers. Most respondents, apparently, want to be "good subjects." This motivation may lead to untruthful responses, especially if interviewees feel that they are being judged by the interviewer. When social desirability and self-presentation are not issues, however, as in cases where the information requested is socially neutral, subjects may be more willing to look to the interviewer for help.

The positive association between accessibility and accuracy has already been discussed. We also found that this relationship was enhanced when the questions involved socially neutral or indeterminate matters, especially when the information had been judged to be relatively inaccessible. That is, questions concerning socially neutral, accessible information generally had high levels of response accuracy. In contrast, responses to questions about socially neutral, inaccessible topics tended to be highly inaccurate.

We assume that respondents are open to reporting socially neutral information if they can remember it, perhaps because this information will not likely occasion self or social judgments. Socially neutral information, however, as compared to that which is negative or positive, may be the most difficult to recall, perhaps because it is not linked in memory to opinions or attitudes concerning social desirability or self-image, or perhaps simply because it lacks specific associates or clearly defined associative networks.

This conclusion suggests that information tied to some affective state, or concerning which an evaluative judgment has been made, may be easier to retrieve than information which simply exists as "data." While we inferred this possibility from our findings, other researchers have reached this same conclusion. Markus (1980), for example, speculated that one of the unique features of self-referent information is that "the self-system is in some way connected with the feeling system or the affective system" (p. 125). Markus further discussed the research finding that the recall of self-referent information is superior to the recall of other types of information. Perhaps the suspected association of affect with cognitions which occurs with self-referent information is at least partially responsible for its greater retrievability. Bower (1981) suggested that the centrality or importance and the distinctiveness of intense emotional events in our lives are the factors responsible for the better recall of these events (for a review of the relevant literature, see Reiser *et al.*, 1985).

Extreme emotionality surrounding an issue may, however, actually block recall. For example, Schacter (1986) noted the "frequently cited relation between extreme emotion during violent crime and claims of amnesia" (p. 289). Freud also concluded that patients resisted recalling emotionally laden experiences that had been repressed or driven out of consciousness. Retrieval of these episodes involving extreme affective reactions to traumatic, threatening events was accomplished only with great difficulty (e.g., Freud, 1909).

Question Topic

That the specific subject matter of the question may be a factor influencing the willingness of respondents to be truthful is widely believed. When we categorized our questions into three groups according to subject, namely, descriptive information and behavior, deviant and personal behavior, and financial matters, and tested the association of the question groups with response accuracy, our findings were inconsistent. We reasoned that question type may affect response validity in a way similar to that of method and question sensitivity. That is, by itself, question content may be relatively unimportant in terms of its influence on response validity. This interpretation leads to two important conclusions. First, as opposed to the specific question content, more attention should be paid to underlying question attributes, such as accessibility. Second, accurate responses can be obtained on a wide range of topics, provided that the questions are crafted and presented with attention to relevant characteristics.

Question Topic and Method

For deviant and personal behavior questions, the use of questionnaires yielded more accurate responses than face-to-face interviews. As previously discussed, questionnaires may allow respondents more time to think through a response. Hesitation is not socially apparent, and respondents may, therefore, be less concerned with being judged or with appearing to be defensive. With questionnaires, respondents may also be more focused on the matter at hand and may have the opportunity to consult other people and records.

Behavioral Prevalence

The direction of the association between behavioral prevalence and response validity varied according to question type category. For questions about descriptive information and behavior, and for questions about financial matters, prevalence and accuracy were positively related. For deviant and personal behavior questions, however, the greater the incidence of behavior performance among the respondents, the lower the level of response accuracy.

These findings suggest that if respondents have engaged in behaviors, they will tend to provide accurate reports about them if possible, at least as they concern descriptive information and behavior and financial matters. In high-prevalence groups, therefore, there are fewer respondents available to report inaccurately. However, when the subject is about personal or deviant behavior, performers may be more motivated to conceal the truth, depending on the interview situation. If there is an overall low incidence of performance of the target deviant or personal behaviors, then most of the respondents can be truthful in their denials.[3]

Summary

The variables that we included in our meta-analyses accounted for a large proportion of the variation in the percentages of accurate responses to the survey questions studied. We found that accuracy tended to be associated

---

[3]We also explored the effect of study date on response accuracy. We tend to conclude that the level of response accuracy has improved over time. Considering that a great deal of attention has been given to this effort over the years, this finding was as expected. There may also be a sociological explanation for this trend, such as an increased tendency to self-disclose, or perhaps a change in perceptions as to what type of information is "private" or under what circumstances disclosure is appropriate.

with certain question characteristics, and that truthful responses could be obtained to questions on a wide variety of topics if the survey questions and conditions helped facilitate information retrieval.

We concluded that for certain types of questions, respondents need time to access the requested information. Particular survey approaches, such as using questionnaires and posing questions in nonbinary formats, may increase accurate responding to those types of questions because they allow respondents to take more time to answer. We were also able to identify questions that might be particularly vulnerable to social influence effects. In those cases, the use of questionnaires was associated with higher levels of accuracy.

A final note: The meta-analysis identified a number of questions that simply cannot be answered because the variables were often highly correlated in the questions we have examined. For example, in our set of general sample questions, sensitive, nonbinary items typically concerned socially undesirable events or behavior. As a result, it was difficult to evaluate one factor independent of another. Some of the questions we have raised will have to be answered by using our analysis as a guide for designing new studies in which the characteristics of the questions are not so highly correlated.

Part V
General Summary

12

Summation and Conclusions

Our two general objectives in this investigation were to assess the degree of response accuracy found in surveys and to identify and systematically evaluate factors which affect response validity. In the past, using a variety of approaches, researchers have attempted to estimate the level of response accuracy to particular survey questions. There has, however, been no previous attempt to pull together the findings from these diverse studies and to systematically and quantitatively analyze the available data.

We concluded that the best approach for our purposes was to examine those survey questions for which the validity of each individual's response had been determined through the use of external criteria. As we examined our data, we identified other issues which we were also able to explore, including the comparison of aggregate-level self-report data with actual figures and whether inaccurate responding is a respondent characteristic or tendency, or related to particular items and item characteristics.

Our results are summarized in detail in the chapter summaries and at the end of each of the major divisions in this report. The qualitative and quantitative examination of the percentages of truthful responses to the hundreds of questions included in our study revealed a large amount of variation in percentages of accurate responses, which occurred both within and across question topic categories and within each of the three major question subsets. Based on our analysis of the questions and the studies, and also considering the speculations of the primary researchers, we identified and discussed certain factors which seemed to have affected response accuracy. In this effort, we were also guided by the literature in cognitive psychology and survey research. A large number of variables that appeared to be influential were then included for evaluation in our meta-analysis.

In the comparisons of self-report with actual data in Chapter 7, we commonly found large discrepancies. Even when aggregate-level estimates were comparable, self-report data often contained serious response errors in the form of over- and understatements, which would make any individual-level assessment of the data problematic.

Particular questions, however, had high levels of response accuracy. This fact suggests differences in question quality in terms of characteristics which facilitate accurate responding. In our research, we have identified and quantitatively assessed many of these question characteristics.

The results of our meta-analysis provided statistical support for certain of the hypotheses generated in the course of our qualitative evaluation of the data. We found that the variables that we included in our quantitative analysis accounted for a large percentage of the variation in response accuracy. We also found that these variables were important to consider not only alone, but in interaction with other question attributes.

Through the meta-analysis, we were able to identify a group of variables that specified question characteristics and survey conditions that either contributed to or detracted from response validity. The single most important factor affecting response accuracy was the accessibility to the respondent of the requested information.

Our results are directly relevant for survey design and survey question construction, because they provide concrete information about question characteristics which affect response accuracy. Our findings may also be useful in evaluating surveys, in estimating survey response validity, and in understanding differences in results across surveys. Additionally, our findings may be of interest to practitioners in other endeavors that depend on self-reports, for example, designing employment applications or obtaining medical and social histories.

We hope that we have provided some insights into the cognitive and social processes underlying respondent behavior. An understanding of these processes, we believe, is essential for developing surveys which will produce valid data.

In addition to its practical value, our research also has theoretical significance. The interpretation of our results was assisted and supported by research and theories mainly from the field of cognitive psychology, but also from social psychology. Gleaned from an analysis of close to 52,000 responses made by individuals from widely diverse subject populations to approximately 250 survey questions over a period of about 40 years, our information will hopefully contribute to knowledge in those fields. Our findings provide research support for certain theories and hypotheses concerning memory and information retrieval. Examples of specific areas which our research may inform are the strategies individuals use when they respond to survey questions and the mental processes involved in the storage and retrieval of information.

That our conclusions were informed by work in cognitive and social psychology, and in turn may contribute to knowledge in those areas, is an example of the type of mutual benefit discussed and encouraged by Loftus *et al.* (1985). Further, that findings from laboratory experiments can be useful in interpreting our results, which are based on data obtained from "real-world" subjects concerning "real-life" behavior and events, demonstrates that research methods with "low ecological validity" (Banaji & Crowder, 1989, p. 1190) can nevertheless have "high generalizability of results" (Banaji & Crowder, 1989, p. 1190).

In attempting to understand and explain our results, we drew on work from a number of areas that we believe may have been previously unrelated, at least in the context of surveys, such as eyewitness identification, social influence, and verbal learning. We hope our work will contribute to the integration of findings from the many diverse areas of psychological investigation.

Motives to distort are often discussed in the survey research literature. In these discussions, the respondent becomes the focus. Our research has led us to focus more on the questions and on the total survey instrument. Our findings suggest that the desire of respondents to be truthful may be greater than commonly believed. For example, our data indicate that inaccuracy is item specific as opposed to being a response tendency on the part of particular respondents across survey questions in general. This finding provides support for the conclusion that it is the question, and associated question characteristics, that prompts or facilitates inaccuracy, as opposed to a motive to distort on the part of the respondent.

Our research also suggests avenues for further investigation. For example, in our report we speculated that certain attributes or conditions were associated with higher levels of accurate responding to particular types of questions because the effect was to provide respondents with more time to consider their answers. The effect on accuracy of providing subjects with more time to respond to these questions needs direct investigation.

Further, we need to determine whether asking respondents questions which call for more than a simple yes or no response results in providing respondents with more time to consider the question. Also, we need to evaluate the comparative accuracy of responses to questions where categories were or were not provided. Other variables that might be included in further investigations include context and type of cues.

We have also noted that researchers have not made full use of the many possible combinations of survey question characteristics. In our meta-analysis, we were not able to examine certain variable interactions due to empty cells or small numbers of cases. Although, for example, we evaluated approximately 150 questions in our analysis of questions directed to general samples, we found no instance where respondents were asked to answer questions concerning descriptive information or behavior with more than a yes or a no. In the future, researchers will hopefully attend to these gaps, perhaps guided by our research and by theories and research in cognitive psychology.

Additional concerns have been expressed about survey data. For example, certain information requested from respondents may simply be unavailable in memory, not just relatively inaccessible. However, in our research, we found that the degree of response accuracy varied according to specific question attributes, suggesting that particular conditions facilitate information retrieval. Information may be available, therefore, but not easily retrievable except under appropriate conditions.

In most aspects of life, it is probably adaptive for individuals to work with generalizations and to have positive beliefs about the self. In survey situations, for accurate responding, respondents may have to engage in unaccustomed behavior, namely, self-reflection. Further, they must use response strategies that are perhaps not commonly used in everyday life. The use of conditions which stimulate these behaviors and strategies promises to increase the accuracy of survey responses.

References

Abelson, R. P. (1981). Psychological status of the script concept. *American Psychologist*, **36(7)**, 715–729.

Asch, S. E. (1951). Effects of group pressure on the modification and distortion of judgments. In H. S. Guetzkow (Ed.), *Groups, leadership and men*, 177—190. Pittsburgh: Carnegie Press.

Baddeley, A., Lewis, V., Eldridge, M., & Thomson, N. (1984). Attention and retrieval from long-term memory. *Journal of Experimental Psychology: General*, **113(4)**, 518–540.

Ball, J. C. (1967). The reliability and validity of interview data obtained from 59 narcotic drug addicts. *American Journal of Sociology*, **72**, 650–654.

Banaji, M. B., & Crowder, R. G. (1989). The bankruptcy of everyday memory. *American Psychologist*, **44(9)**, 1185–1193.

Bauman, K. E., Koch, G. G., & Bryan, E. S. (1982). Validity of self-reports of adolescent cigarette smoking. *International Journal of the Addictions*, **17(7)**, 1131–1136.

Begin, G., & Boivin, M. (1980). Comparison of data gathered on sensitive questions via direct questionnaire, randomized response technique, and a projective method. *Psychological Reports*, **47(3)**, 743–750.

Bekerian, D. A., & Bowers, J. M. (1983). Eyewitness testimony: Were we misled? *Journal of Experimental Psychology: Learning, Memory, and Cognition*, **9(1)**, 139–145.

Blaney, P. (1986). Affect and memory: A review. *Psychological Bulletin*, **99(2)**, 229–246.

Bower, G. H. (1981). Mood and memory. *American Psychologist*, **36(2)**, 129–148.

Bradburn, N. M., Rips, L. J., & Shevell, S. K. (1987). Answering autobiographical questions: The impact of memory and inference on surveys. *Science*, **236**, 157–161.

Brown, R. (1986). *Social psychology: The second edition*. New York: The Free Press.

Brown, R., & McNeill, D. (1966). The "tip of the tongue" phenomenon. *Journal of Verbal Learning and Verbal Behavior*, **5**, 325–337.

Cahalan, D. (1968). Correlates of respondent accuracy in the Denver validity survey. *Public Opinion Quarterly*, **32**, 607–621.

Cannell, C. F., & Fowler, F. J. (1963). A comparison of a self-enumerative procedure and a personal interview: A validity study. *Public Opinion Quarterly*, **27**, 250–264.

Cannell, C. F., & Kahn, R. L. (1968). Interviewing. In G. Lindzey & E. Aronson (Eds.), *The handbook of social psychology* (2nd ed.). Reading, MA: Addison-Wesley.

Clancy, K. J., Ostlund, L. E., & Wyner, G. A. (1979). False reporting of magazine readership. *Journal of Advertising Research*, **19(5)**, 23–30.

Clark, J. P., & Tifft, L. L. (1966). Polygraph and interview validation of self-reported deviant behavior. *American Sociological Review*, **31**, 516–523.

Clark, J. P., & Tifft, L. L. (1967). Reply to DeFleur. *American Sociological Review*, **32(1)**, 115–117.

Clausen, A. R. (1968). Response validity: Vote report. *Public Opinion Quarterly*, **32(4)**, 588–606.

Crossley, H. M., & Fink, R. (1951). Response and non-response in a probability sample. *International Journal of Opinion and Attitude Research*, **5(1)**, 1–19.

Cutler, B. L., Penrod, S. D., & Martens, T. K. (1987). The reliability of eyewitness identification. The role of system and estimator variables. *Law and Human Behavior*, **11**, 233–258.

David, M. (1962). The validity of income reported by a sample of families who received welfare assistance during 1959. *Journal of the American Statistical Association*, **57**, 680–685.

Diener, R., & Wallbom, M. (1976). Effects of self-awareness on antinormative behavior. *Journal of Research in Personality*, **10**, 107–111.

Elffers, H., Vrooman, J. C., & Hessing, D. J. (1985). Non-experimental research in economic psychology: A field study of fiscal behavior. *Proceedings of the Tenth International Association for Research in Economic Psychology Annual Colloquium*.

Elffers, H., Weigel, R. H., & Hessing, D. J. (1987). The consequences of different strategies for measuring tax evasion behavior. *Journal of Economic Psychology*, **8(3)**, 311–337.

Erickson, M. L., & Empey, L. T. (1963). Court records, undetected delinquency, and decision-making. *Journal of Criminal Law, Criminology, and Police Science*, **54**, 456–469.

Ericsson, K. A., & Simon, H. A. (1980). Verbal reports as data. *Psychological Review*, **87(3)**, 215–251.

Ferber, R., Forsythe, J., Guthrie, H. W., & Maynes, E. S. (1969a). Validation of a national survey of consumer financial characteristics: Savings accounts. *Review of Economics and Statistics*, **51**, 436–444.

Ferber, R., Forsythe, J., Guthrie, H. W., & Maynes, E. S. (1969b). Validation of consumer financial characteristics: Common stock. *Journal of the American Statistical Association*, **64(326)**, 415–432.

Freeman, H. (1953). A note on the prediction of who votes. *Public Opinion Quarterly*, **17**, 288–292.

Freud, S. (1909). Five Lectures on psychoanalysis. Translated and edited by James Strachey (1977). New York: Norton.

Glass, G. V. (1976). Primary, secondary, and meta-analysis of research. *Educational Researcher*, **5(10)**, 3–8.

Gottfredson, M. R., & Hindelang, M. J. (1977). A consideration of memory decay and telescoping biases in victimization surveys. *Journal of Criminal Justice*, **5**, 202–216.

Gray, P. G. (1955). The memory factor in social surveys. *Journal of the American Statistical Association*, **50**, 344–363.

Groves, R. M. (1989). *Survey errors and survey costs*. New York: Wiley.

Hagburg, E. C. (1968). Validity of questionnaire data: Reported and observed attendance in an adult education program. *Public Opinion Quarterly*, **32**, 453–456.

Hardin, E., & Hershey, G. L. (1960). Accuracy of employee reports on changes in pay. *Journal of Applied Psychology*, **44**, 269–275.

Hardt, R. H., & Peterson-Hardt, S. (1977). On determining the quality of the delinquency self-report method. *Journal of Research in Crime and Delinquency*, **14**, 247–257.

Hasher, L., & Griffin, M. (1978). Reconstructive and reproductive processes in memory. *Journal of Experimental Psychology: Human Learning and Memory*, **4(4)**, 318–330.

Hawkins, D. I., & Coney, K. A. (1981). Uninformed response error in survey research. *Journal of Marketing Research*, **18(3)**, 370–374.

Hessing, D. J., Elffers, H., & Weigel, R. H. (1987). Exploring the psychology of tax evasion behavior: Personality, reasoned action and the limits of self-reports. (draft).

Hessing, D. J., Elffers, H., & Weigel, R. H. (1988). Exploring the limits of self-reports and reasoned action: An investigation of the psychology of tax evasion behavior. *Journal of Personality and Social Psychology*, **54(3)**, 405–413.

Horvitz, D. G. (1974). Discussion. *Proceedings of the Social Statistics Section of the American Statistical Association*, 28–29.

Hyman, H. (1944). Do they tell the truth? *Public Opinion Quarterly*, **8(4)**, 557–559.

Ito, R. (1963). An analysis of response errors: A case study. *Journal of Business*, **36**, 440–447.

Kassin, S. M., Ellsworth, P. C., & Smith, V. L. (1989). The "general acceptance" of psychological research on eyewitness testimony: A survey of the experts. *American Psychologist*, **44(8)**, 1089–1098.

Katosh, J. P., & Traugott, M. W. (1981). The consequence of validated and self-reported voting measures. *Public Opinion Quarterly*, **45(4)**, 519–535.

King, J. D., Lewis, H. S., & Rogers, C. B. (1981). The problem of respondent recall: A note on the consequences of using inaccurate survey data. *Political Methodology*, **7(2)**, 1–12.

Kinsey, K. A. (1984). *Survey data on tax compliance: A compendium and review.* Taxpayer Compliance Project Working Paper 84–1. Chicago: American Bar Foundation.

Kinsey, K. A. (1988). *Measurement bias or honest disagreement? Problems of validating measures of tax evasion.* Chicago: American Bar Foundation Working Paper 8811.

Lansing, J. B., Ginsburg, G. P., & Braaten, K. (1961). *An investigation of response error.* Urbana, IL: University of Illinois, Bureau of Economic and Business Research.

Latane, B., & Darley, J. M. (1970). *The unresponsive bystander: Why doesn't he help?* New York: Appleton-Century-Crofts.

Light, R. J., & Pillemer, D. B. (1984). *Summing up: The science of reviewing research.* Cambridge, MA: Harvard University Press.

Locander, W. B., Sudman, S., & Bradburn, N. (1976). An investigation of interview method, threat, and response distortion. *Journal of the American Statistical Association*, **71**, 269–275.

Loftus, E. F., Fienberg, S. E., & Tanur, J. M. (1985). Cognitive psychology meets the national survey. *American Psychologist*, **40(2)**, 175–180.

Loftus, E. F., & Palmer, J. C. (1974). Reconstruction of automobile destruction: An example of the interaction between language and memory. *Journal of Verbal Learning and Verbal Behavior*, **13**, 585–589.

Long, S. B., & Swingen, J. A. (1991). Tax compliance: Setting new agendas for research. *Law & Society Review*, **25**, 637–683.

Malbin, J. H., & Moskowitz, J. M. (1983). Anonymous versus identifiable self-reports of adolescent drug attitudes, intentions, and use. *Public Opinion Quarterly*, **47(4)**, 557–566.

Markus, H. (1980). The self in thought and memory. In D. M. Wegner & R. R. Vallacher (Eds.), *The self in social psychology*. New York: Oxford University Press.

Mauldin, W. P., & Marks, E. S. (1950). Problems of response in enumerative surveys. *American Sociological Review*, **15**, 649–657.

Maynes, E. S. (1965). The anatomy of response errors: Consumer saving. *Journal of Marketing Research*, **2**, 378–387.

McFarland, S. G. (1981). Effects of question order on survey responses. *Public Opinion Quarterly*, **45(2)**, 208–215.

Midanik, L. (1982). The validity of self-reported alcohol consumption and alcohol problems: A literature review. *British Journal of Addiction*, **77(4)**, 357–382.

Milgram, S. (1974). *Obedience to authority*. New York: Harper.

Miller, H. P. (1953). An appraisal of the 1950 census income data. *Journal of the American Statistical Association*, **48**, 28–43.

Miller, M. (1952). The Waukegan study of voter turnout prediction. *Public Opinion Quarterly*, **16**, 381–398.

Myers, D. G. (1990). *Social psychology* (3rd ed.). New York: McGraw-Hill.

Myers, D. G., & Ridl, J. (1979). Can we all be better than average? In D. Goleman & D. Heller (Eds.), *The pleasures of psychology*. New York: New American Library.

Nelson, D. L., Bajo, M. T., & Casanueva, D. (1985). Prior knowledge and memory: The influence of natural category size as a function of intention and distraction. *Journal of Experimental Psychology: Learning, Memory, and Cognition*, **11(1)**, 94–105.

Nelson, D. L., & Friedrich, M. A. (1980). Encoding and cuing sounds and senses. *Journal of Experimental Psychology: Human Learning and Memory*, **6**, 717–731.

Nisbett, R. E., & Wilson, T. D. (1977). Telling more than we can know: Verbal reports on mental processes. *Psychological Review*, **84(3)**, 231–259.

Parry, H. J., & Crossley, H. M. (1950). Validity of responses to survey questions. *Public Opinion Quarterly*, **14(1)**, 61–80.

Popham, R. E., & Schmidt, (1981). Words and deeds: The validity of self-report data on alcohol consumption. *Journal of Studies on Alcohol*, **42**, 355–358.

Reder, L. (1987). Strategy selection in question answering. *Cognitive Psychology*, **19**, 90–138.

Reiser, B. J., Black, J. B., & Abelson, R. P. (1985). Knowledge structures in the organization and retrieval of autobiographical memories. *Cognitive Psychology*, **17**, 89–137.

Robins, L. N. (1966). Deviant children grown up: A sociological and psychiatric study of sociopathic personality. Baltimore: Williams and Wilkins.

Rogers, T. F. (1976). Interviews by telephone and in-person: Quality of responses and field performance. *Public Opinion Quarterly*, **40**, 51–65.

Rosenberg, M. J. (1968). Hedonism, inauthenticity, and other goads toward expansion of a consistency theory. In R. P. Abelson, E. Aronson, W. J. McGuire, T. M. Newcomb, M. J. Rosenberg, & P. H. Tannenbaum (Eds.), *Theories of cognitive consistency: A sourcebook*. Chicago: Rand McNally.

Rosenthal, R. (1978). Combining results of independent studies. *Psychological Bulletin*, **85(1)**, 185–193.

Ross, L. D., Amabile, T. M., & Steinmetz, J. L. (1977). Social roles, social control, and biases in social perception processes. *Journal of Personality and Social Psychology*, **35**, 485–494.

Schacter, D. L. (1986). Amnesia and crime: How much do we really know? *American Psychologist*, **41(3)**, 286–295.

Seltzer, R. (1983). Sponsorship effects in an attitudinal survey. *Political Methodology*, **9(4)**, 447–452.

Singer, E., Frankel, M. R., & Glassman, M. B. (1983). The effect of interviewer characteristics and expectations on response. *Public Opinion Quarterly*, **47(1)**, 68–83.

Skogan, W. G. (1981). *Issues in the measurement of victimization.* U.S. Department of Justice, Bureau of Justice Statistics.

Smith, K. W. (1974). On estimating the reliability of composite indexes through factor analysis. *Sociological Methods and Research*, **2(4)**, 485–510.

Smith, K. W. (1988). *Will the real noncompliance please stand up? Complexity and the measurement of noncompliance.* Paper presented at IRS Research Conference, Washington D.C.

Sobell, L., & Sobell, M. (1978). Validity of self-reports in three populations of alcoholics. *Journal of Consulting and Clinical Psychology*, **46**, 901–907.

Sobell, M., Sobell, L., & Samuels, F. (1974). Validity of self-reports of alcohol-related arrests by alcoholics. *Quarterly Journal of Studies on Alcohol*, **35**, 276–280.

Spanier, G. B. (1976). Use of recall data in survey research on human sexual behavior. *Social Biology*, **23(3)**, 244–253.

Sudman, S., & Bradburn, N. (1974). *Response effects in surveys.* Chicago: Aldine.

Thomson, D. M., & Tulving, E. (1970). Associative encoding and retrieval: Weak and strong cues. *Journal of Experimental Psychology*, **86(2)**, 255–262.

Tittle, C. R., & Hill, R. J. (1967). The accuracy of self-reported data and predictions of political activity. *Public Opinion Quarterly*, **31**, 103–106.

Tulving, E. (1985). How many memory systems are there? *American Psychologist*, **40(4)**, 385–398.

Tulving, E., & Pearlstone, Z. (1966). Availability versus accessibility of information in memory for words. *Journal of Verbal Learning and Verbal Behavior*, **5**, 381–391.

Tulving, E., & Thomson, D. M. (1973). Encoding specificity and retrieval processes in episodic memory. *Psychological Review*, **80(5)**, 352–373.

Tversky, A., & Kahneman, D. (1974). Judgment under uncertainty: Heuristics and biases. *Science*, **185**, 1124–1131.

Udry, J. R., & Morris, N. M. (1967). A method for validation of reported sexual data. *Journal of Marriage and the Family*, **29**, 442–446.

Voss, H. L. (1963). Ethnic differentials in delinquency in Honolulu. *Journal of Criminal Law, Criminology, and Police Science*, **54**, 322–327.

Weaver, C. N., & Swanson, C. L. (1974). Validity of reported date of birth, salary, and seniority. *Public Opinion Quarterly*, **38(1)**, 69–80.

Weiss, C. (1968). Validity of welfare mothers' interview responses. *Public Opinion Quarterly*, **32(4)**, 622–633.

Wilkins, A. J. (1971). Conjoint frequency, category size, and categorization time. *Journal of Verbal Learning and Verbal Behavior*, **10(4)**, 382–385.

Wonnacott, T. H., & Wonnacott, R. J. (1977). *Introductory statistics for business and economics* (2nd ed.). New York: Wiley.

Yaniv, I., & Meyer, D. E. (1987). Activation and metacognition of inaccessible stored information: Potential bases for incubation effects in problem solving. *Journal of Experimental Psychology: Learning, Memory, and Cognition*, **13(2)**, 187–203.

Zajonc, R. B. (1965). Social facilitation. *Science*, **149**, 269–274.

Index

ISBN 0-12-744030-5

90065